Mediterranean And Ketogenic Lifestyle

Sidney Collar

Contents

Chapter One

INTRODUCTION

WHAT THE PROTEIN DIET IS AND HOW TO DO IT

People who consume a diet high in protein and low in carbs tend to lose weight faster, according to several doctors and nutritionists. A diet high in protein and low in carbs has been found to help eliminate the indications of heart disease and allow the pounds to just melt away, according to well-known institutions, such as the Mayo Clinic.

So, what exactly is a protein diet, and is the routine it necessitates really worth it? Many believe it is the solution to the obesity epidemic and a way for people to retrain their eating habits for a healthier lifestyle. Some people have been able to postpone or avoid gastric bypass surgery by following this eating regimen.

Should You Be Eating More Protein?

People who follow a high-protein diet report feeling fuller longer. Because of their high protein content, meats including chicken, turkey, fish, and even hog are included in the diet. The original diet has undergone various iterations, some of which include carbohydrate restriction and warning or attack phases. However, this is not your typical low-carbohydrate diet. This diet differs from others in that it focuses on protein rather than carbs.

Most low-carbohydrate diets do not need calorie tracking. One must not only count calories but grammes of protein in this strategy. The protein level of every food a person consumes must be closely controlled. Excess protein intake without adequate calories can be hazardous, even fatal. Because of this, this diet plan demands a set quantity of calories in addition to the right amount of protein. Depending on a person's weight loss goals, they have varying demands.

What about the healthy foods like vegetables and fruits?

Of course, this plan incorporates certain aspects of a carbohydrate-based diet. Even the simplest fruit, such as an orange, is high in carbs, which are harmful to your health. This diet plan instructs a person to consume meals that contain less carbs and are more filling in order to avoid hunger and provide the body with the fuel it needs. For example, strawberries, honeydew, watermelon, and raspberries all have lower carbohydrate content than bananas or apples. This is because to the fruit's high water content. Carbohydrates are reduced when fruit is more watery.

Carbohydrate content in vegetables is low to non-existent. Potatoes, sweet potatoes, maize, and carrots are the only common vegetables to be omitted from this diet. All other veggies may normally be eaten in whatever quantity desired by the individual. The body won't want sweets as much if you eat a diet rich in veggies. Starch is abundant in potatoes, and starch is converted to sugar in the body. This diet's core tenet is to limit carbs and increase protein intake. Fiber and protein grammes are more important than calorie count when choosing a protein source. Some vegetables, such as spinach, provide the body with more nutrients than others, such as carrots.

Protein and plant-based foods are prominent in the diet.

Where Would We Be Without Protein?

Meat is only a small portion of the total amount of protein that may be consumed by a human being. Eggs, beans, nuts, legumes, and meat can all be eaten. Pork can be eaten, however it should be avoided if it is heavily fatty. The objective is to consume at least 200 grammes of protein every day. When following a classic low-carbohydrate diet, a person does not count the grammes of protein or fat in their food.

On a low-carbohydrate diet, it doesn't matter how much fat is in the meat; but, on a high-protein diet, leaner cuts are prefered.

To ensure a well-balanced diet, this strategy reduces fat consumption as well as a small number of calories. Is there a standard amount of protein in most foods? For example, a can of tuna has roughly 100 grammes of protein, but the body requires more than simply protein to function properly.

Tuna is a low-calorie food, therefore it should be paired with other options that are part of the overall diet plan.

This Diet Plan Is Used By Whom?

Weight-loss dieters and bodybuilders should follow a high-protein diet plan. Because of its immediate outcomes, it helps those who are overweight to bring their weight under control more quickly. Detoxification is accelerated by the increase in protein and decrease in sugar intake. The body will be able to burn stored fuel more quickly when it removes all the sugar from its system. First-week weight loss can be as high as 6 to 10 pounds for those who follow this plan's "induction or assault phase." Metabolic jump-starting and weight reduction are both aided by this.

It's well-known that losing weight happens swiftly. Reintroducing breads and other carbohydrate-rich meals might lead to weight gain if the proper quantities are not taken, so be cautious. The body goes into famine mode when it is deprived of glucose. The body will begin to use fat reserves as a source of energy when in this state. As you can see, the end effects are very remarkable. People on this diet lose an average of 1-2 pounds a week.

Do You Have to Follow This Diet?

Losing weight rapidly is something that the entertainment industry is always on the lookout for new diets and trends to try. The low carbohydrate diet has benefitted many, but declaring that one should never again consume bread or fruit is overly pessimistic as well. Bananas and oranges are inevitable cravings for everyone. The purpose of this diet is to increase protein intake while decreasing carbs and fat intake, with the hope of achieving significant results.

Chapter Two

MY PERSONAL ADVICES

WHERE TO FIND PROTEIN IN YOUR DIET

Weight reduction is a common goal for those on protein-rich diets. A high-protein diet combined with regular exercise, according to some experts, can help people lose weight. Protein-rich diets also aid in the preservation of lean body mass by allowing the body to burn fat for energy.

In order for the body to operate correctly, one must consume enough amounts of protein. Growth, strength, and weight loss are just few of the health advantages that this mineral provides. A wide variety of protein-rich foods are available to consumers. Protein drinks and bars are popular with many individuals. Hypotension and anaemia are only a couple of the illnesses that can be brought on by a lack of protein in the diet. Muscle mass might deteriorate and result in fatigue if protein intake is inadequate. Diets strong in protein and low in carbohydrates have long been popular. There are several ways to lose weight on a protein-rich diet. Listed below are a variety of various protein diets.

The Atkins Diet is a popular weight loss plan.

Dr. Robert Atkins developed the Atkins Diet, which is a weight-loss strategy. Meat, poultry, fish, and eggs are all acceptable sources of protein and fat in this diet, which also limits the use of starchy vegetables like maize, peas, and potatoes and allows for the consumption of oils and butters. This low-carbohydrate diet claims that you will lose weight and that you will not feel hungry.

Among other health benefits, this diet promises to improve cognition and cardiovascular health.

People who are overweight are advised by the Atkins diet to reduce their carbohydrate intake. When it comes to generating energy, the body uses both carbs and fat, but carbohydrates take precedence over fat. Eating more protein and fat helps the body shed pounds because it burns fat more quickly when less carbs are consumed. Weight loss, excellent health, and illness prevention are all claimed by the Atkins diet.

The Zone Diet

The Zone Diet was developed by Dr. Barry Sears. The Zone Diet allows dieters to eat a wide variety of foods, but they must adhere to the prescribed calorie and macronutrient ratios. The Zone Diet promotes frequent, low-calorie meals as a means of losing weight. Canola, olive, avocado, and macadamia nuts are all part of the Zone diet. There are several foods that are restricted on the Zone Diet, such as pasta, bread, and some fruits. Glucose is easily released from these carbs, which is why they are limited. To put it simply: The Zone Diet has more protein and fat per unit of weight than other diets.

Diet of the South Beaches

The South Beach Diet was developed by Dr. Arthur Agatston. In order to follow this diet, one must follow a method called the glycemic index. The meals in this diet are ranked based on how quickly their sugars reach the bloodstream. In comparison to other protein-based diets, the South Beach Diet is said to be healthier since it allows for the eating of whole grains, lentils and beans, low-fat dairy products, vegetables, and good fats from nuts and fish, as well as fats such as olive oil Carrots and fruits, which have a high glycemic index, are prohibited on the South Beach Diet.

There are various phases to the South Beach Diet. The induction phase, which lasts for the first two weeks, is designed to help dieters overcome their cravings for carbs. As a result of this, carbs are kept to an absolute minimum in the diet. High-processed carbohydrate meals, according to the South Beach Diet, are absorbed too rapidly. Insulin levels rise as a result of this. Insulin is a hormone that the body secretes to aid in the breakdown of sugar.

An increase in insulin levels when carbs are depleted causes a person to seek additional food. Someone will eat if this occurs.

extra sugars and starches The South Beach Diet is designed to assist dieters in breaking the pattern of overeating and encouraging them to eat fewer, but higher-quality, amounts.

The Power of Protein Diet

Drs. Michael and Mary Eades developed the Protein Power Diet. All forms of meat, poultry, fish, eggs, butter, non-starchy vegetables, oil, cheese, and salad dressing are encouraged on the Protein Power Diet. Alcohol is permitted in moderation on this diet as well.

Grains, starchy vegetables, fruits, and milk are all restricted on this diet.

This low-carbohydrate eating plan, like other low-carbohydrate diets, is built on the premise that managing insulin levels can assist manage a variety of blood parameters, including triglycerides and insulin resistance. A high amount of insulin inhibits the breakdown of fatty deposits in the body, which is caused by the consumption of carbohydrates. On the other hand, decreased carbohydrate consumption is associated with higher concentrations of insulin.

As a result, weight loss occurs. Fat melts away if you keep doing this for a long time.

The Stillman diet

The Stillman Diet was established by Irwin Maxwell Stillman. Many decades have passed since the original formulation of this high-protein, low-carbohydrate diet. When compared to the Atkins diet, which restricts carbohydrates, the Stillman Diet restricts fat consumption. This diet has a lot of protein in it. Lean proteins like skinless poultry, lean meat, eggs, fish, seafood, and low-fat cheese are promoted as well as lean sources of protein whereas sources of oil, fat, and carbs such fruits, vegetables, breads, and pastas are restricted.

a low-sugar diet

Moderate alcohol intake is permitted together with low-glycemic meals such as all proteins and fats. White rice, potatoes, bread, carrots, beets, maize, and other refined white flour items are all off limits on the Sugar Busters Diet. Whole grains, vegetables strong in fibre, lean and trimmed protein, fruits, and fish are the mainstays of the diet. Red wine is the best choice if you want to drink alcohol. Cook meat on the grill, in the oven, or on the broiler, and use oils that are high in mono- and polyunsaturated fats and low in saturated fats. Moderate-sized meals should be had three times a day. It is okay to have a snack like almonds or fruit on this diet, however the fruit should be eaten on its own.

Considerations

Weight reduction can be achieved by a high-protein, low-carbohydrate eating plan. Some people may not be able to handle high-protein diets. Before embarking on a high-protein diet, you should get the advice of your doctor. Moderate calorie consumption and increased physical activity are the best ways to reduce weight, according to experts. There are several diet and exercise programmes out there that can help you lose weight and become in shape. Set your priorities and stick to them.

DUKAN DIET - WHAT IS IT?

In the Dukan Diet (also known as the French Protein Diet), weight loss is encouraged and proposed via the use of natural methods. Dr. Pierre Dukan, a French nutritionist, invented it more than a decade ago and aimed it at obese individuals. The Dukan Diet incorporates a healthy eating plan. This diet includes 72 animal-based items and 28 plant-based foods.

The Attack Phase, the Cruise Phase, the Consolidation Phase, and the Stabilization Phase make up this diet plan.

As many "excellent foods" as the dieter desires are allowed to be consumed on the diet. If you compare the Dukan Diet to other weight loss regimens, you'll notice that there is no calorie tracking or food rationing.

People can eat as much of the things on the list as they wish as long as they follow the guidelines. For this diet, protein is the most important component. Both the Dukan and Atkins diets emphasise protein as a key component of their diets. The Atkins diet, on the other hand, allows for the consumption of fat.

There are 72 different high-protein and low-fat items to choose from during the assault phase, which is the first part of the diet. A person is unable to consume anything else throughout this period. Water, coffee, and tea are the only beverages permitted during this period. Dietary choices include everything from low-fat steak to fat-free cottage cheese during the first phase. Additionally, oat bran can be consumed throughout this time period. Exercise plans like a 20-minute stroll every day are used by some dieters. For the past five days, I've been on a five-day protein diet. People who have gone through the assault phase claim to have lost seven to ten pounds in only five days. The assault phase lasts only a few seconds and ends with immediate fulfilment.

During the cruise phase, you alternate between days when you simply consume protein and days when you consume both protein and veggies. Like phase 1, oat bran can be included into the second step. In this period, dieters can walk for 30 minutes at a time. Optional protein and vegetable days can be substituted for the more restrictive protein ones, or vice versa. This person might alternate between a 5-day protein and vegetable fast followed by a 4-day protein-only fast. During the voyage period, there are only a few veggies available to eat.

Because some vegetables are high in carbs, they are banned from the diet. Most green vegetables, including asparagus, celery, and green beans, are permitted. For some dieters, this phase might last for many weeks or even months, depending on how much weight they hope to lose.

The Dukan Diet's consolidation phase, which lasts 10 days per pound lost, is the third and final phase. This phase may only be entered when the desired weight has been achieved. It helps dieters maintain their weight loss by teaching them how to eat a healthy, balanced diet once they reach their goal weight. While there is some latitude, it is closely checked to ensure that the desired weight is not strayed from. Even if you've lost a lot of weight, you're still at risk of putting it all back on again if you're not careful. Two celebratory dinners (or feasts) are served throughout this time period.

Celebration meals (to encourage a gradual return to the food that is sought) are offered in order to promote a gradual return to eating. It is now OK to eat fruit, cheese, and bread in moderation.

They can have one fruit every day, but they must be watery ones (i.e. apples and cantaloupe). Wholegrain bread can also be consumed every day. Each week, dieters are only permitted one portion of carbs and one special occasion meal. After shedding a lot of weight, you'll need to maintain that weight reduction in order to avoid regaining it. During this time, participants should not expect to lose weight; instead, they should focus on returning themselves to a healthy diet.

The final step, stability, is the fourth phase. This is the most critical stage, since the majority of dieters regain the weight they lost throughout the diet. As a starting point, dieters should utilise the phase 3 diet to guide their food choices. To keep the weight off, one should adhere to the guideline of having one day a week dedicated solely to protein intake. Dieters are said to be able to eat anything they want at this period.

This, however, is the most common blunder made by dieters. Dieters who revert to their former eating patterns will see their weight creep back on. In this period, dieters should proceed cautiously while keeping an eye on what they eat. As previously said, while choosing meal selections, the preceding three stages should be utilised and taken into account. As a dieter, it's in your best interest to keep up your exercise routine.

The Dukan Diet 100 Eat As Much As You Want Items" is the name given to the foods that are included in this diet. Meat, poultry, fish, seafood, eggs, dairy products, vegetables, and vegetable proteins are all included in this dietary group. Increasingly popular, the Dukan diet has been translated into 10 languages, making it available to a global audience. As of this writing, the product is available in more than 20 countries. According to reports, 5 million individuals in France have allegedly lost weight using it.

It's a safe and effective way to shed pounds that won't come back. Carbohydrates and lipids are severely restricted, whereas proteins are given first priority. Maintaining a healthy diet and lifestyle is essential for everyone. There is a lot of evidence that this diet works. Before embarking on any diet or exercise regimen, it is important to visit a doctor to confirm that it is safe.

The DUKAN ATTACK-PHASE ONE DETAILED.

The Dukan diet is a four-step plan that teaches you how to eat healthfully and shed pounds. Pierre Dukan, a French physician, developed the method to assist obese people lose weight quickly. Over five million individuals in France lost weight on the diet. The Dukan diet is now available in the United States, thanks to celebrity endorsements attesting to its effectiveness. It's a low-calorie, high-protein diet that promises to help you lose one pound a day.

As many as ten pounds have been reported to have been lost by many during the assault phase. The Dukan assault is the initial part of the process that will lead to a new you. A single meal should not be equated with the entire diet. There are four phases: the attack phase, which is followed by the cruise phase, consolidation phase, and stabilisation phase. While each step of the diet has its own importance, I will focus on the assault phase, which is the most critical.

A total of 72 distinct varieties of food are available to you throughout this period. These meals are high in protein, low in fat, calories, and carbs. Being that this list comprises primarily of animal products like meat and seafood, it's sure to be a hit with meat and seafood lovers everywhere! As long as you keep to this category of foods, you can eat as much as you like. You must, however, keep one thing in mind throughout this stage. Only one-half teaspoon of oat wheat bran per day is permitted in your daily diet. During the assault phase of the diet, this oat bran keeps you full. There are several sorts of meals that you may consume, including lean beef and veal as well as shellfish, eggs, and low-fat dairy items. There is no restriction on how you consume them as long as you stick to this category.

Seasoning your cuisine with herbs and spices is OK. You may also season your meats and seafood with lemon, zest, and garlic.

Anything that makes you happy and keeps you on track to achieving your goals Roasted or grilled meats and fish are also suggested as a fat-free alternative to frying. From 5 to 10 days, you might continue this phase of the attack.

How much weight you desire to reduce is a determining factor.

In order to avoid becoming tired with eating the same thing over and again, there are several recipes available to help you experiment with different food combinations. A sugar hunger can be soothed with fat-free yoghurt or jello, both of which contain no sugar at all. After a time, you'll find yourself thinking, "Cinnamon roll what?" after eating so many of them. Once you know how beneficial a healthy diet is to your health, it ceases to be a key focus.

When it comes to drinking, your selections in the beverage category differ somewhat from those available in the food category. When it comes to food, you have a lot of alternatives, but when it comes to beverages, you have a limited selection.

Everyone knows that water is the healthiest beverage to consume, therefore that is the primary selection you have. It is necessary for you to take 1.5 cups of water.

A quart of water every day. A cup of coffee or tea is counted against your daily water intake, even if you don't drink it. Adding a cup or two of coffee or tea to your water intake gives people who aren't used to drinking so much water a choice. When it comes to your health, drinking plenty of water is critical since it aids digestion, aids in hydration, and promotes a faster metabolism. In addition, it is important to note that sugar is not permitted in your coffee or tea. For people who need their coffee or tea to be sweetened, the best option is to stay with water.

This diet has little to no adverse effects. Constipation and/or bad breath from the bath are possible side effects. However, sugar-free gum or 1 1/12 teaspoon of oat wheat bran, both of which include fibre, can help prevent these problems.

This diet does not need you to engage in any physical activity. It's possible that exercising during the attack phase might help you lose weight more quickly and build muscle. A twenty minute stroll has never damaged anybody.

Some people may ask if this diet is good for you. With that said, it's not hard to see that the meals you're currently eating are healthy ones. You're eliminating all of the unhealthy stuff from your diet and replacing them with healthy ones. Things like fruits and veggies will ultimately be included in as you progress through the rounds. During this phase, you'll learn how to ditch your bad eating habits and replace them with healthier ones, all while losing a significant amount of weight.

You need to stick to the plan that has been meticulously laid out for you to follow. If you make a mistake, you may have to start again from scratch. You will be thrown off course the moment you puncture the diet, as mentioned by the designer himself. Staying on track is essential if you want to lose the weight you want to lose.

PHASE TWO OF THE DUKAN DIET CRUISE DISCOVERED

The Dukan Diet is one of the most popular and effective diets currently available. Obesity has become a serious public health issue in the United States, Europe, and throughout the globe. In order to lose weight, many people have tried the Dukan Diet to help them achieve their goal weight. There are four phases to the Dukan Diet, which are the Attack, Cruise Consolidation, and Stabilization phases.

Before long, when you've completed the Attack Phase and gained a thorough understanding of its strength, you'll be on your way to completing the Cruise Phase. This part of the diet is a lot of fun, since you can eat whatever you want and not feel restricted in any way. You've made it through the Attack Phase, lost a few pounds, and now you're ready to go for your goal weight. The Dukan Diet is one of the most adaptable weight-loss plans available, making it a realistic goal for most people.

In order to begin the Cruise Phase, you must have completed the Attack Phase by losing a significant amount of weight. All of your favourite meals were removed from your diet during the Attack Phase and replaced with high-protein, low-carbohydrate options. As a result, you shed pounds quickly, but at a rate you can't keep up. During the Cruise Phase, you'll learn how to regulate your body's metabolism so that weight loss occurs more gradually and over a longer period of time.

The Dukan Diet's Cruise Phase is based on a philosophy of strict discipline. Using an easy-to-maintain diet, you'll teach your body new ways to eat and operate. You'll be eating more veggies during the Cruise phase than you did during the Attack phase.

It is recommended that you alternate days of consuming pure protein foods and those that include veggies in your diet throughout the Cruise Phase. Turkey burgers, fat free yoghurt, salmon and eggs might be included in a pure protein day. Instead of yoghurt on a pure protein day, celery sticks with a low-fat dip might be a snack on a day where you combine protein with veggies. Potatoes are the only vegetable you cannot eat at this time because of their high carbohydrate content.

The major goal of this alternate diet is to provide your body with a steady supply of protein and veggies while yet allowing you to lose weight gradually and steadily. This diet is expected to result in a two-pound weight loss each week. Even if you have a cheat day or an off day, you still want to make sure that your weight is constantly trending in the right direction and that you are making progress.

So, how about some physical activity while you're in the Cruise Phase? During the Dukan Diet's second phase, you'll be doing more exercise. During this time, it is expected that you would walk for at least 30 minutes every day. This is a step up from the Attack Phase, which focuses more on accelerating your metabolism. Your muscles will grow as a result of this additional exercise as well as your ability to burn calories. Increased exercise will help build the lean muscle mass needed to shed those extra pounds because muscle burns fat.

So, how long do you stay on the Dukan Diet during the Cruise Phase? This phase of the diet has no specified time limit. You'll be on this diet for a long time, unlike the Attack Phase, which only lasts for seven days. Once you have reached your goal weight, the diet's "cruise phase" will be over. So, if your goal weight is 160 pounds and you are now 180 pounds, you must maintain your diet until you reach your weight loss goal. As a result, if necessary, the Cruise Phase may extend for an additional month or months. Again, we're all realistic enough to realise that no diet is going to be flawless all the time. If you're determined to reach your ideal weight, you'll get there.

Dukan Diet Cruise Phase, if you're looking to have the most fun, is it. During this time, you have the freedom to try new protein-based dishes and protein-vegetable combos. To begin, experiment with different meal plans and switching between protein and vegetables on different days of the week to see what works best for you. Try some of the Dukan Diet's best-known dishes, such as chicken chilli, turkey chilli, and seafood paella, for example. If you gain a pound or two in a week, don't freak out. Just take a look back at your eating habits for the week and determine if it was due to inactivity, an excess of carbs, or some other factor. You'll be able to make adjustments and keep moving towards your goal weight.

When it comes to losing weight, it doesn't have to be an all-out war. You can get the weight you've always wanted if you eat a diet rich in protein and veggies. The Cruise Phase might be the most difficult and time-consuming part of the Dukan Diet since it forces you to focus on exactly what you are putting into your body. However, your body will appreciate you after you manage your diet and learn to eat in new, better ways. When you reach your goal weight and are ready to begin phase three of the diet, the Consolidation Phase, you will be rewarded.

EXPLAINED: PHASE THREE OF THE DUKAN DIET CONSOLIDATION PROCESS

Even though dieting requires a great deal of self-control, many people find it difficult to maintain their weight loss once they've achieved it. Consolidation-Phase Three of the Dukan Diet explains how to gradually reintroduce foods to your body. After going on a diet, many people discover that they either overeat or completely disregard their dietary restrictions. Using the Dukan Diet Consolidation-Phase Three Explanation, dieters may begin a more gradual transition to eating less and eating more often.

This diet eliminates binge eating, allowing your body to gradually adapt to a more natural method of consuming food, preventing a sudden weight gain.

When thinking about nutrition, it is vital to keep things in perspective. It's very uncommon for dieters to eat their way back into their weight-loss struggles, but this is no longer the case for those following the Dukan diet.

This diet forbids the consumption of certain items. Slim and trim, your weight is moving in the way you want it to. It's challenging to go out to dine with friends when you're on a restrictive diet, but it's possible. Lamb, duck, lentils, and dairy products are all items to steer clear of if you're trying to lose weight. In general, stay away from high-fat foods. These are items that most people avoid, making your transition to a new diet easier. During the consolidation phase, your body gradually emerges from its slumber. As a result of your efforts to limit your intake of fattening foods, your body is now prepared to re-enter the world of eating with a new set of abilities and knowledge.

This is the first weight loss approach that some users have found that also helps them control their cravings for food. A Dukan Diet participant's physique can only improve as a result of their efforts in the gym, water consumption, and calorie tracking. Other people are envious of your success and wonder how you managed to become so strict with your diet.

Consolidation is indicated for a maximum of 50 days, depending on how much weight the individual has lost.

It's difficult not to overeat while you're on or trying to go off a diet. The digestive system suffers when food is consumed too rapidly. Gradual progress is preferable if done carefully. Adding a few carbs to your diet during the Consolidation or Phase 3 Stage is perfectly OK. During this period, take a moment to admire your development in the mirror. Take a moment to notice how good you feel.

Exercise isn't on the agenda, but you'll start doing it once you see how much better you look in clothes you couldn't wear before. There is a lot less effort involved in implementing this method of progressive meal introduction.

Cherries and bananas are prohibited in this sector, which requires a moderate amount of protein and some fruit. Some whole grain bread slices and some cheese are included in the list of things to do. If you're a big fan of cheese, this may be a wonderful treat. During the first portion of this diet, you are allowed one serving of starchy food, while in the second portion, you are allowed two servings of starchy food. Keep in mind that this is only a stepping-stone to consuming normal meals.

Pastas, potatoes, and lentils are all included in the menu. Until recently, these items were absolutely prohibited for dieters to consume. They're back, but in moderation, for the time being. Seasoning is allowed on this diet, so long as you don't overdo it. Cooking with herbs is a lot of fun since they can enhance the flavour of even the most bland of liquids. In this phase, lentils are permitted; if you add more seasoning, the meal becomes highly flavorful..

As the process progresses, more and more delicious foods are making a come-back. It's OK to have lamb, but greasy eating isn't part of the experience. Now that you've changed your eating habits, you're ready to learn about the Dukan Diet Consolidation-Phase Three. Treat yourself to a nice dinner during the first half of the consolidation period. This makes even the most difficult situations tolerable. When you achieve a goal, treat yourself to a meal you like. After that, treat yourself to another reward supper, but this time, resist the urge to overindulge. Don't let go of the self-control you've gained via dieting. It's a wonderful thing to get rid of harmful habits.

Eat protein for the duration of this adjustment phase. Eat a little amount of oat bran every day. Take two tablespoons of the mixture and add it to the bowl. Drinking a lot of water is a no-brainer. This is a critical step in the consolidation process. Add a little amount of walking to your workout routine, and you'll notice a noticeable difference in your physique. Toning is necessary for any weight loss you've achieved. You'll put your control over your eating habits to the test in this phase. It's beneficial for your health, and it'll get you moving. Taking a walk will help alleviate any concerns you may have about overeating. People's days may be made or broken by food, and if that's the case for you, this portion of the diet can help you regain some control.

It's a victory when one can break free of a bad habit. It's hard to say no to food at holidays, weddings, and family gatherings because of the abundance of it. This diet teaches you how to control your food consumption, but it's a gradual process. This can't be overstated. Make a budget for your food. It's almost the same. When you overindulge, your body suffers.

Dukan Diet Consolidation-Phase Three Explained has shown to be an effec-tive weight loss method for many people.

Learning to eat healthfully is an ongoing process, and this diet helps you navigate each step. Since you won't be starved throughout the Consolidation Phase, there's no need to get too hungry. However, it doesn't provide you with enough to jeopardise your growth.

Stabilization-PHASE FOUR OF THE DUKAN DIET IS DETAILED.

There are four stages of the Dukan diet. Stabilization is the name given to the last stage. It's at this point in the low-fat, high-protein diet that the dieter must put an end to their weight loss and take charge of their destiny. The most important thing is to follow the guidelines to the letter. The final phase of lifetime transformation is the fourth phase.

Phase Four: What Is It Good For?

The Dukan diet's fourth phase aims to help you sustain your new eating habits by reducing limitations while also enhancing your sense of personal responsibility. Simple and easy-to-follow eating habits are the goal of these alterations. The most critical thing to keep in mind is that this is the stability phase of the diet. Now that the hard work is done, it's time to make sure the progress made in the previous phases stays on track. Now that they've gotten to this phase, you're free to eat however you normally would. You must, however, continue to consume meals that are rich in nutrients.

However, there is a significant difference between the third and fourth phases. The fourth phase, in contrast to stages two and three, is more permissive.

What are the Dukan Diet's Phase 4 benefits?

The Dukan Diet is based on the idea of consuming a lot of protein but very little fat throughout the day. Increased muscle mass and decreased intake of calories and bad cholesterol are the goals of this diet. In the end, you'll have a more athletic and slim body. The final phase of the procedure is phase four. In this phase, the major advantages are a sense of accomplishment and a reduced number of rules. Efforts to finish have been made. You need to grab life by the horns and commit to a healthy lifestyle. This may be achieved by a balanced diet and regular physical activity.

Phase Four Diet Portion - What Is It?

In order to maintain weight reduction throughout the Dukan Diet's fourth phase, you must take extremely particular dietary measures. These activities, on the other hand, are quite simple to use. For the most part, you are free to eat anything you want. When it comes to eating, there are a few rules to keep in mind. The majority of these recommendations will be based on the prior phase's guidelines. Protein must be the primary component of your diet, regardless of what else you eat. Nuts, beans, seeds, and lean meats are all healthy choices. Vegetables are fine to eat. Fruit should be had just once a day, whereas wholegrain bread should only be consumed twice a day.

A carb-heavy dinner might be eaten once a week if you so choose. Once a week you can have pasta, for example.

One to two dinners a week are the highlight for many folks. Anything you may think of can be included in these customised dinners.

eat. However, it is essential that this type of food be had just on certain times. This meal does not count if it occurs to be in accordance with the regular limits in any manner. If a person eats anything that isn't from one of the permitted food groups, it is considered a special meal. However, there is a one-of-a-kind regulation. Every week, at least one meal must be made entirely of protein. That day, there can be no other form of food.

Phase Four of the Dukan Diet Requirements for Exercise

The Dukan Diet allows for a wide variety of workout options. This diet won't work without it. You must engage in physical activity on a daily basis and to the level necessary to enhance your capacity for self-motivation. The assumption that expending calories genuinely aids in weight loss is the driving force behind this decision.

Every day, you must at the very least go for a vigourous walk. It will begin with a 20-minute walking session, but it will gradually increase. This time limit will rise to 30 minutes when the phases of the diet are completed. The weight will fall more rapidly if you exercise with a goal in mind. In order to maintain your weight loss, you'll need to work out every day in phase four. The most effective way to shed pounds is through a combination of diet and exercise. This is the only set of tools you'll ever need.

Please keep in mind that the recommended amount of walking is merely a bare minimum. The health advantages of resistance training and weight lifting are far bigger than the benefits of brisk walking on a daily basis. In addition to walking, which is a great all-around workout, there are specialised training methods that may help you lose weight and build muscle.

Considerations at the End of the Road

Please see a doctor before starting this diet. Many of the food types you're used to eating will be off limits on this diet. For a period of time, this might lead to nutritional shortages while you learn new eating habits and discover healthy substitutes for the foods you were used to consuming.

In spite of the fact that a low-fat and carbohydrate diet has been success-fully completed, it might nevertheless cause weariness. Constipation, mood changes, and strange bodily sensations are all things to keep an eye out for. It is expected that these concerns will be resolved over time.

It is possible to suffer from headaches and bad breath if you consume a big amount of protein on a regular basis. This diet requires that you consult your doctor if you have a medical condition. For example, if you have kidney disease, you should not follow this diet at all.

Some dieters find this plan appealing since it permits them to eat artificial sweeteners and diet Coke while on it. Note that none of these things are nutritionally sound and may even be hazardous to your health in the long run.

Recipes from the DUKAN DIET

Tandoori-Spiced Lemon Roasted Chicken

15 minutes of prep time

Depending on the size and weight of the bird, 1 12 to 2 hours should be allotted for baking

These are the ingredients you'll need: (Serves 2)

1 chicken, entire

A sugar-free tandoori spice blend of 7 tablespoons

a quarter of a lime

Directions:

Set the oven temperature to 350 degrees.

Open up the skin of the chicken's breast so that lemon slices may be inserted into it. Add 3 teaspoons of tandoori spice and 4 slices of lemon to the opening.

Keep doing this until you get two pouches over the chicken's legs. Each cavity should be filled with a slice of lemon and two pieces of cheese.

Spices from the tandoori oven.

Roast the chicken for 1 12 to 2 hours, or until it reaches an internal temperature of 165 degrees Fahrenheit, in a roasting pan set on the middle oven rack. Using a knife, cut into the thickest section of the chicken until clear liquid flows from the cavity.

Serve immediately after removing the skin.

All Spiced Salmon

5 minutes of preparation time

Depending on the size of the fillet, the baking time is around 20 minutes.

These are the ingredients you'll need: (Serves 2)

The two huge salmon fillets

ground black peppercorns

all-spice in 1 teaspoon

Directions:

To get started, preheat the oven to 350 degrees and prepare a baking sheet with parchment paper. Infuse the flesh with the taste of the salmon skin by making diagonal slices.

Place salmon fillets skin side up on the tray. Spice and pepper each cut liberally.

Bake the fish fillets for about 20 minutes, until they reach an internal temperature of 135 degrees and the skin begins to crisp, then remove them from the oven.

Indian Omelet with a Spicy Kick

These are the ingredients you'll need: (Serves 1)

2 hens' eggs

1 Tbsp. Olive Oil

6 chopped green chilis, with seeds removed

half a thinly chopped red onion

1 finely minced spring onion.

Diced fresh coriander is all that is needed for this dish.

Just a pinch of garam masala

Some turmeric, please!

In a nutshell:

Directions:

In a medium-sized bowl, whisk together the eggs and the rest of the ingredients. Add olive oil to an 8-inch nonstick pan and heat it to medium.

The bottom should start to set after a few minutes of slowly pouring in eggs. Lift the omelette, allowing the extra liquid to flow beneath. Before folding, cook for a few more minutes.

Tuna and Egg Green Beans

5 minutes of preparation time

10 to 20 minutes of cooking time

These are the ingredients you'll need: (serves 2)

1 cup fresh green beans, drained and rinsed

2 hens' eggs

2 tins of tuna fish

The minced garlic of one clove

Salt

Directions:

Garlic and green beans should be steamed for around ten minutes (or to desired texture). Make a pot of boiling water for the eggs.

Eggs should be peeled and chopped. Add tuna, eggs, and salt to green beans and mix well.

Gnocchi with oat bran Dukan

5 minutes of preparation time

5 minutes of cooking time

These are the ingredients you'll need: (Serves 1)

1 12 to 2 tbsp. oat groats

0.01% of an egg

1-teaspoon yoghurt

1 tbsp. of fresh cheese

Directions:

Combine the fromage frais, oat bran, and quark in a bowl and whisk until well combined.

Beat the egg whites to a stiff froth, then fold them into the batter. Olive oil should be added to a nonstick pan that is heated to medium-high heat.

Pour the ingredients into the blender in a steady stream. Cook for 2 to 3 minutes on each side.

Rolls of Chicken with Pesto Sauce

These are the ingredients you'll need: (serves 1)

1 cup of chunked chicken breast

2 crepes made with oat bran

Basil leaves, finely chopped

2 tbsp. of extra virgin olive oil

Garlic, minced into 1 clove

Chunks of dried sun-dried tomato

Directions:

In order to make pesto out of basil, garlic, and olive oil, simply combine the ingredients.

Cooked chicken breasts.

Layer chicken and tomatoes on the crepes and wrap them up with a toothpick before serving.

Salad of Mackerel Smoked in the Oven

10 minutes of preparation are required.

About 6-8 minutes of hands-on time

These are the ingredients you'll need: (Serves 1)

fillet of sablefish (smoked)

1 cup florets of broccoli

Two cherry tomatoes, each cut in half

Spinach leaves in a cup (baby)

Alfalfa sprouts in a quarter-cup serving

Half of a red pepper sliced

1 tsp. mustard powder

1 tbsp. of cooking oil

14 tsp. white vinegar (white wine)

Directions:

To cook the mackerel, follow the directions.

Broccoli should be steamed before being rinsed and drained under running water (cold).

Chop up and toss all of the vegetables except for the spinach and the tomatoes.

Put the mackerel in the salad and chop it up. The oil should be combined with the other ingredients and whisked until smooth. The salad should be drizzled with a mixture of white wine vinegar and mustard.

Butternut squash, turkey, and curry

15 minutes of preparation time

Cooking time: twenty-five minutes.

These are the ingredients you'll need: (Serves 4-6)

Peel and slice a small onion.

Garlic, minced into 1 clove

1 tbsp. of finely sliced peeled ginger

a pinch of korma powder or curry powder

Coriander leaves, about a half cup

peel and slice one red onion

12 pound of sliced turkey breasts

1 12 pounds of diced up butternut

1 pound of baby spinach

1 tbsp. corn starch

a tablespoon of soy sauce

2 teaspoons of sweetness

Some low-fat yoghurt (about 2 tablespoons)

Directions:

Put ginger, garlic, onion, korma spice, and coriander leaves in a blender and process until smooth.

2-3 minutes of cooking time in a big pan should do the trick.

1 34 cups of water, the curry paste, and the butternut squash go into the pot. Begin heating up. Simmer for 15 minutes or until butternut is fork-tender. Reduce heat.

Add the spinach and toss well to combine the flavours. Make a paste out of the maize flour, soy sauce, sugar, and half a cup of water by mixing them together. Add to the curry paste and continue stirring until it thickens to your desired consistency. Serve with a dollop of yoghurt on top.

Background Information about the Writer

Healthy nutrition has always been a priority for Louise A. Costas. When it comes to diets, she wants to know everything about what they promise to do and what, if any, consequences they may have. She's aware that fad diets come and go, so she doesn't fall for them. Instead of focusing on whether or not a diet would be simple to stick with, she is concerned that it will need too much of an effort on her part.

To avoid making unnecessary modifications and giving up on the diet altogether, she typically does not even bother starting one in this second case. For this reason, she's looking for diets that are easy to follow so that she can adhere to them and eventually reap the benefits. It will be a great read for you if you agree with her sentiment.

Diabetic Ketosis

To transform your fat into lean muscle, follow a diet low in sugar and starch.

7 Days Of Energy

WHAT IS THE KETOGENIC DIET?

A ketogenic diet consists of a high-fat, low-carbohydrate, high-protein intake. It was originally designed as a specific diet for children with epilepsy. This diet provides just enough protein each day to support development and repair. In order to keep the child's weight in line with their height and weight, the appropriate number of calories must be delivered.

History

The Mayo Clinic created the ketogenic diet in 1924. In his research, Dr. Russel Wilder discovered that placing epileptic patients on a fast reduced the frequency of their seizures. This is the ratio of fat to protein and carbohydrate in the traditional diet, which is 4:1.

Avoiding foods heavy in carbohydrates should be a priority while trying to lose weight. Starchy vegetables, fruits, cereals, pasta, and sugar are all examples of high-carbohydrate foods.

Anticonvulsant medications have lowered the popularity of this diet as a technique of managing epilepsy. The stringent ketogenic diet was a challenge for most patients and health care providers. The Johns Hopkins Medical Center and a few other medical facilities still offer and employ the diet as a therapy option.

It wasn't until the mid-1990s that the ketogenic diet was resurrected as an effective treatment for epilepsy. As a child, Jim Abrahams had a two-year-old son who was diagnosed with epilepsy. The ketogenic diet was a part of the child's recovery. It was shown that following this diet helped to reduce or eliminate the seizure activity. The Charlie Foundation was established by the family as a result of their achievement. It contributed to the study of the ketogenic diet. In 1997, First Do No Harm, a made-for-television movie, helped raise awareness of this diet as a therapy option. In the years afterwards, there has been an increase in scientific interest in nutrition and its prospective applications.

What are the underlying principles of a keto diet?

A daily carbohydrate intake of 20 to 50 grammes is recommended.

Moderate protein consumption is seen. It varies according on the gender, height, and activity.

To maintain a healthy weight, a person should consume a healthy amount of fat in relation to their overall caloric intake.

The following is a typical breakdown of calories:

o 70% to 80% of the daily calories are fat.

· 20% to 25% of the protein

The carbohydrates in food make up between 5% and 10% of the total weight of the product.

In order to induce and maintain ketosis, a certain ration of foods is used.

What's the deal with the ketogenic diet's higher proportion of fat and lower proportion of protein?

Insulin and blood sugar levels are unaffected by fats.

If you eat a lot of protein, your insulin and blood sugar levels might be affected. As a result, the ketogenic diet suggests consuming it in moderation.

A whopping 56% of the extra protein we consume is transformed into simple sugars. When the body responds to the glucose generated by protein breakdown, the ketosis state of fat burning will be disrupted.

Rabbits can starve to death if their diets are low in fat and protein.

o Fat deficiency is one of the causes of rabbit hunger. Lean protein-heavy diets are more likely to have this problem. Diarrhea is the most concerning sign, as it has the potential to become life-threatening. Diarrhea usually develops within the first three to seven days after starting a diet high in lean protein. Diarrhea develops and might lead to dehydration and mortality if appropriate fats are not included in the following days.

Eating a lot of fat has been shown to improve health. The kind and origin of fat are important considerations. Saturated fats, together with minimal carbohydrate intake, help to enhance the body's fat composition. Trans fat levels are reduced while HDL (the "good" cholesterol) is up. People who have this sort of fat profile are more protected from heart attacks and cardiovascular disease.

What is the mechanism through which the diet functions?

The ketogenic diet is designed to put your body into a state of ketosis. Carbohydrates are the first fuel that the body tends to utilise. Carbohydrates are the most readily absorbed and digested of all macronutrients. When carbs are depleted, the body turns to fats and proteins for energy. When it comes to the way the body uses energy, there is a hierarchy. Carbohydrate is first used by the body when it is accessible.

Next, the body turns to fats for energy. The final stage of protein conversion into energy happens when the body is starved of carbs and fat reserves have already been exhausted. Muscle wasting is caused by the body's digestion of the proteins found in muscles.

Ketosis is a natural state of affairs for the body. During fasting, this occurs. As an illustration, consider the time spent dreaming. It is common for the body to burn fats for energy during sleep while the body heals and expands.

Carbohydrates account for the majority of the calories in a typical meal. Carbohydrates are more likely to be used for energy and stored as fat and protein (i.e., fats and proteins). Many calories come from fat rather than carbs while following a ketogenic diet. When following a ketogenic diet, you consume very little carbohydrate, which is quickly burned off. There is an apparent "energy shortage" as a result of the reduced carbohydrate intake. The body then turns to the fats it has stored as fuel. It transforms from a carbohydrate-to-fat converter. Fats from the recent meal are not immediately utilised, but are saved until the next phase of ketosis, which begins after the next meal. Because fat-burning has become a normal mode of obtaining energy, the body uses up all of the fat in the most recent meal, leaving a small amount for storage.

A large fat intake on the ketogenic diet is therefore necessary to meet the current energy needs and save some for the future. During periods of fasting, stored fat is critical in preventing the body from breaking down muscular protein reserves. These intervals in a day's cycle are quite natural. Sleep and the time in between meals are also called fasting times. At these moments, the body still requires a continual flow of energy. In the absence of fat reserves, the body will turn to the proteins stored in the muscles for energy. A high-fat diet can help prevent this from happening.

In order to replicate starving state, the ketogenic diet is the most important aspect. As a result, the body is deprived of quick-digesting carbohydrates that can be readily transformed into energy. The body is compelled to enter fat-burning mode as a result.

As a bonus, it increases the production of fat-mobilizing hormones such as catecholamines, cortisol, and growth hormones. The ketosis state, or fat-burning mode, is triggered by this trio of hormones.

Ketosis and Ketones in Chapter 2

When following a ketogenic diet, your body goes into a state of ketosis. After a decline in blood glucose levels, the body uses fat as a source of energy. The fat that has been accumulated in the body is burned to provide energy. Ketones are byproducts of the body's fat metabolism. The carbonyl functional group connects two atom groups in these molecules. The cells can utilise them as a source of power. About 70 to 75 percent of the brain's energy needs can be met by ketones.

Ketosis Is Induced By...

The body goes into a ketotic condition when the cells are depleted of glucose. To meet the body's glucose requirements, there aren't enough carbs. In the following circumstances, ketosis is induced:

• Dehydration and malnutrition

When you're starving or fasting, your body isn't getting enough food to digest and turn into glucose. During sleep, fasting, or missing meals, the body goes into starvation mode. Low blood glucose levels are caused by a lack of meal consumption. The stored glucose in glycogen is released. In order to provide the body with energy, they are transformed into glucose. Body fat is burned to help the body convert glucose into energy. When one is in a ketotic condition, ketogenesis takes place (lack of available glucose). This is the process through which fats are metabolised to create ketones, a kind of alternative energy.

• Insulin-related issues.

• Moderate carbohydrate consumption

Ketosis's impact on the human body

When you're in ketosis, your body produces and excretes ketones. There are a few symptoms that might be both good and bad as a result of these chemicals.

Effects That Aren't Positive

As the body becomes accustomed to using ketones for energy, the majority of the side effects fade away. By the end of the first week after beginning a ketogenic diet, the majority of people have adjusted. Others might take up to two weeks. Up to 12 weeks may elapse before the body is fully used to the fat-burning regimen.

The desired outcomes frequently take longer to manifest. Between 6 and 8 weeks, subtle benefits can be observed.

Lack of strength

a feeling of dizziness or faintness

• Tiredness.

• Pain in the head

• A tinge of irritation

high levels of triglycerides (if too much unhealthy fats)

Throwing up

• Diabetic ketoacidosis

Only if the body's control mechanisms malfunction may this impact occur. In the absence of insulin, the ketone levels rise.

that's already potentially harmful to your health. Ketoacidosis is the medical term for this illness. Ketosis produced by nutrition, on the other hand, is insufficient to bring on this state.

Ketogenic diets can be used to treat children with epilepsy. Some of the documented adverse effects of this diet are as follows:

Irritation of the Stomach

• The loss of water

• Stones in the kidneys or gallbladder

• Growth that has slowed or stopped altogether

• a feeling of slumber

An increase in gastroesophageal reflux symptoms

Bruising is more common.

Fractures are more likely to occur as a result of this.

• Ketosis and acidosis in excess

"Psychosocial" non-consumption

Women with epilepsy who follow a ketogenic diet report the following side effects:

• Mood swings throughout the menstrual cycle

Concerns about the eyes

Loss of bone mass

Pancreatitis

The limits have the potential to lead to deficits in micronutrients. Carbohydrate-heavy diets are often packed with vitamins and minerals.

Deficiencies in these vital nutrients may result from the extreme limitations on carbohydrate consumption. Micronutrient (vitamin and mineral) consumption and macronutrient (fat, protein, and carbohydrate) counts and proportioning in meals are critical. In order to avoid deficient conditions, supplementation may also be required.

Uses of the Ketogenic Diet in Chapter 3

As a result, the body transforms into a fat-burning machine rather than one dependent on carbohydrates. A high-carbohydrate diet has been related to insulin resistance and diabetes, according to research.

Absorption and storage are both easy with carbohydrates. The mouth is where digestion begins. As soon as the food is eaten, salivary amylase (an enzyme that breaks down carbs) begins working. As soon as carbs enter the small intestines, they're broken down and absorbed. Carbohydrates instantly raise blood sugar levels in the bloodstream. Insulin is released right away as a result of this. Insulin levels increase when blood sugar levels are high. To reduce blood sugar levels, this hormone allows glucose to be stored in the body's tissues right away. Insulin resistance can develop in tissues that are repeatedly exposed to high doses of the hormone. Overconsumption of carbs leads to weight gain and obesity.

This loop can lead to diabetes and cardiovascular disease.

Certain medical disorders have been proven to benefit from a high-fat, low-carbohydrate diet known as a ketogenic diet. As part of the therapy strategy, it is necessary.

Epilepsy

When on a ketogenic diet, epileptic seizures appear to be less frequent. The ketogenic diet was developed for this same purpose. Patients with paediatric epilepsy respond well to this kind of diet. Even after a few years of following the ketogenic diet, some children have completely eliminated their seizures. Adult epilepsy responds poorly to treatment.

A few days of fasting may be necessary before starting the ketogenic diet for epilepsy therapy.

Cancer

Ketogenic dieting has been shown to put cancer into remission, according to current studies. In order to alleviate the symptoms, it "starves cancer."

disease of the brain in people with Alzheimer's

A ketogenic diet has been shown to improve cognitive function in Alzheimer's disease patients. They are able to restore some of their mental and memory abilities.

Diseases of the brain

Neurological illnesses including Parkinson's disease and ALS (amyotrophic lateral sclerosis) benefit from a ketogenic diet. Mitochondria are supported in nerves that are impacted by the diet. As a result, the symptoms are alleviated.

Diabetes

Diabetes is mostly caused by an excess of carbohydrates in the diet. Blood sugar levels are more easily managed when the ketogenic diet is restricted. This diet can be used in combination with other diabetic treatment strategies.

An intolerance to certain grains

There are a lot of people who aren't aware that they have a gluten allergy. Symptoms such as bloating and intestinal pain improved after following a ketogenic diet. Most carbohydrate-rich meals have a significant amount of gluten. It is also possible to reduce gluten consumption by removing many carbs from the diet. There are no longer any issues with gluten.

Loss of weight

There is a growing market for the ketogenic diet. The fact that it has been shown to have the side effect of encouraging weight reduction has led to its inclusion in many dieting plans. At first, many people were sceptical of the concept of shedding pounds on a high-fat diet. Weight reduction programmes are gradually adopting the ketogenic diet because of its more positive effects over time.

Carbohydrates, not lipids, are the primary cause of weight gain. Remember that insulin encourages the accumulation of carbs, which leads to weight gain. It is possible to lose a significant amount of weight by reducing or eliminating carbohydrate intake.

Which Foods Are Prohibited?

Ketosis is mostly induced by limiting carbohydrate intake. In spite of this, our bodies are capable of adapting to a new diet. As a result, controlling protein and fat intake is essential.

Fats

A ketogenic diet tends to emphasise the consumption of fats. During the ketosis state, it is the primary source of energy. Fats should account for 60 to 80 percent of daily caloric intake. The value varies according to the diet's objective. Epilepsy sufferers may consume as much as 90% of their daily caloric intake from lipids.

But there are a few rules to follow when deciding which fats to incorporate.

• There are no polyunsaturated omega-6 fatty acids in this product. Large levels of omega-6 fats have been shown to be inflammatory.

– Corn oil.

– Soybean paste

– Cottonseed Oil

Inflammatory omega-6 fatty acids can be found in seed and nut oils, which should be avoided.

- Oil of almonds

Oil made from flaxseed

- Seed oil from sesame

Do not use commercial salad dressings, such as mayonnaise, on your salads. If you can't avoid it, check the carbohydrate content.

Avoid trans fats and hydrogenated fats. They've been connected to an elevated risk of heart disease and other cardiovascular issues.

Proteins

The choice of proteins is critical since it has long-term consequences for the diet. The use of steroids and antibiotics in animals has the potential to induce health issues in humans. Grass-fed, organic, and free-range are the best options. Avoid animals that have been given hormones, especially rBST.

The carbohydrate level of the extenders or fillers employed might be a deciding factor when it comes to processed meat purchases. Beef cured with honey or sugar should be avoided.

Carbohydrates

Carbohydrates are severely restricted on a ketogenic diet. Depending on the individual's activity level and metabolic rate, the limitation is determined.

Carbohydrate consumption on the ketogenic diet is often limited to fewer than 50 or 60 grammes per day. Carbohydrates can be consumed as much as 100 or more grammes per day by those with a healthy metabolism and those with greater metabolic rates (like athletes).

People with Type 2 diabetes who are sedentary may need to limit their daily carbohydrate intake to no more than 30 grammes. Whether or whether you can handle it depends on your tolerance level and your overall health. In addition, the goal of a ketogenic diet must be taken into consideration.

Vegetables:

Ketogenic diets rely heavily on vegetables for their carbohydrate content, although some should be avoided. Peppers, tomatoes, and onions are some of the veggies that contain a lot of sugar. The majority of subterranean vegetables are starchy, carrying a high amount of carbs.

Sweets

Because they contain a lot of sugar and carbs, normal sweets should be avoided at all costs. These are the names of them:

When it comes to cakes,

• Cakes, pastries, and other baked goods

Bread & buns •

The glistening sugar of fruit

Diet chocolate and other chocolate varieties, such as lollipops, are included in this category.

• Biscuits: plain, filled with cream, iced, or chocolate-covered

• Pastries

Pâtisseries and other sweet treats

Puff Pastries

• Syrups and icings with added sugar

• Condensed whey

desserts like ice cream

All forms of jam, including diabetic jam, are included.

• Flavorings of milk

• Drinks such as Ovaltine, Milo, and Quik are all examples of chocolate-based concoctions.

• Dishes

• Chutneys and pickles

Maltodextrin or some other kind of sugar may be present in the artificial flavouring used to flavour flavoured yoghurt.

• Sweetened beverages like sodas and alcoholic beverages like alcoholic beverages.

• Juice from fruit

Do not swallow any sugarless gum.

• Cough syrups and drugs that have been sweetened.

Sugars

Glucose is abundant in sugar, which is why it should be avoided. Brown sugar, white sugar, castor sugar, and icing sugar are some of the more common varieties of sugar. It can also be found in processed foods and pharmaceuticals as a medicine additive.

FOODS PERMITTED IN THE CAMP

Ketogenic diet meals are mostly composed of three fundamental food kinds. A fruit or vegetable, a protein-rich meal, and a fat source are all included.

Fats

The ketogenic diet necessitates an increase in fat intake. They may be used in the same way as frying pans and pan grills are. Sauces and dressings can also include fats. Another simple approach to include fats in your diet is to butter a piece of steak before eating it.

When it comes to the greatest sort of fat, you should stick to ketogenic ones. Oils with medium-chain triglycerides, such as MCT oil and coconut oil, are prefered. Ketones are easily produced by the metabolism of these lipids.

Ketosis-friendly fats include the following:

Fats with fatty acid ratios of 3:6:3

It's all about the fish, right?

- Sockeye

- Tuna is an excellent source of protein.

- Crabs and shrimp

mono- and polyunsaturated fatty acids

Olive oil

It's red palm oil.

— The word "butter"

— CHEESE

— Acai berries

- The yolks of eggs

Unrefined and unrefined oils (when cooking)

- Tallow from beef

— Lards without hydrogenation

- Using coconut oil is a great way to keep your skin

oleic acid content is high.

- Oils made from safflower

Sunflower oils

Other sources of fat include:

- Peanut butter is an excellent source of protein.

- The skin of chicken is included in this.

- Meats with a lot of fat on them

- Butter from coconut

Proteins

The ketogenic diet allows for the consumption of any sort of meat. No matter what style of cut or preparation, it does not discriminate.

Pork

Beef

veal

Venison is an excellent source of protein.

• A suckling pig

The term "poultry" encompasses all forms of poultry. The fat content of the meal is higher when the skin is left on, thus it is recommended that you do so. Breading and batter should not be used in preparation since they contain a lot of carbohydrates. Individual taste dictates what constitutes an acceptable preparation.

• Poultry

There are several species of quail.

• Turkey, on the other hand, is a

• Oysters

In addition to meat and poultry, fish and seafood are excellent sources of protein. The omega-3 fatty acids, vitamins, and minerals in some of these foods can aid in the maintenance of healthy

fed and in good health

• Seafood

Omega-3 fatty acids are found in abundance in fish. Choose wild-caught fish that has not been exposed to mercury.

- Tuna is an excellent source of protein.

Caught in the act

Fish – Halibut

- The Flounder

Coho

— Mahi-mahi fish

In other words, Snapper.

It's all about the fish, right?

- Sockeye

- Mackerel is the fish of choice.

• Seafood

- Clams on the half shell

the Squid

the delectable shellfish

As for the crab, –

– Crab

'Mushrooms'

- Scallops are a delicacy in this country.

Carbohydrates

• Fruits and Vegetables. •

For carbs, the ketogenic diet relies mostly on vegetables. You can't go wrong with organically cultivated produce. Organic and non-organic foods have similar nutritional values. The difference is in the danger of eating vegetables that have been sprayed with a fungicide or other chemical. The lowest carbohydrate concentration is seen in dark leafy vegetables, which are also high in nutritional value.

Leafy greens, such as spinach

- Aquatic Plants and Flowers

- All kinds of cabbage.

A wide variety of lettuces are available.

In this case, the Kale

- Brussel sprouts are an excellent source of vitamin C.

Bok Choy

Celery –

- Cucumbers. –

- Cauliflower is an excellent source of vitamin C.

– Sprouting beans

– Radishes.

The vegetable known as Asparagus

• Dairy Products and Milk

A ketogenic diet would be incomplete without milk and dairy products. Preference is given to natural and organic products. Full-fat options are preferable to fat-free or low-fat alternatives.

When it comes to the keto diet, eggs are a must have. It is an excellent source of both protein and fat.

- Different kinds of cheese, both hard and soft. Carbohydrates are present. Carbohydrates from cheese should be included in your daily intake. Here are a few examples:

o Mascarpone cheese

I'm talking about Cheddar.

This is a Mozzarella

Yes, I'm talking about cream cheese.

the aforementioned dairy product, cottage cheese

It's also a good idea to incorporate sour cream in your diet. As a result, the food has a richer, more varied flavour.

There are a number of different types of nuts.

Nuts can be eaten in moderation on a ketogenic diet. They provide a lot of protein, fat, and carbs, which is good for you. Keto diets should contain nut varieties that have been evaluated for their carbohydrate, fat, and protein contents. Nuts and seeds roasted to perfection and

In order to go into ketosis, seeds are the greatest option since they eliminate anything that might be harmful or interfere with it.

- Snacking on nuts is one of the most common ways to consume them.

Almonds, macadamias, and walnuts are the best nuts to incorporate.

– Omega-6 fatty acids, which are abundant in certain nuts, have the potential to promote inflammation in the body.

- Cashews and pistachios have more carbs. These should be stacked with care.

• Herbs, spices, and condiments

It's normal to find it tough to get used to eating less carbs during the first few weeks of a ketogenic diet. Those with a sweet taste may find it difficult to control their urges. Pasta and processed foods, which are heavy in carbohydrates, might be dull and unappetising to those who consume them often. After a while, eating just ketogenic meals might get monotonous. Spices may provide a dash of flavour. Spices, both fresh and dried, can be added to food and drinks to enhance flavour and intrigue the senses.

Carbohydrates can be found in spices. There should be a daily carbohydrate and ketogenic count for even a few.

Added sugars are common in pre-made spice blends. To get an exact count of the overall carbohydrate count, read the labels.

Salt can be used to improve the flavour. Sea salt is better than table salt since it doesn't include dextrose powder. Ketogenic dieters should stay away from this form of sugar.

Spices may be used for more than simply taste; they can also provide a number of health advantages. These are a few of the healthful spices:

"Baby"

— Peppercorns.

Peppercorns from the Cayenne plant

– Coriander

- Cinnamon is a flavouring ingredient.

In a nutshell:

– Cumin

Leaf parsley

- Oregano is a great addition to any dish.

- Sage's words

Rosemary: –

A spice called turmeric

A savoury herb, thyme

Sweeteners

The use of artificial sweeteners can help alleviate cravings for sugar and carbs. They aid in sticking to the ketogenic diet and attaining success. Stevia and E-Z Sweets are the finest artificial sweeteners. In terms of the carbohydrate count, they have no effect.

Because no binders like dextrose and maltodextrin were used, liquid sweeteners are preferable. The following sweeteners come highly recommended:

- Sucralose is a sugar substitute (liquid form is recommended)

As a sugar substitute, xylitol is an excellent choice.

- Erythritol is a sugar substitute.

the Monk fruit —

Beverages

Dietary restrictions on carbohydrates cause the body to excrete waste products through the kidneys and bladder. Water retention occurs as a result of carbohydrate absorption. Reduced carbohydrate intake causes water retention and increased water excretion. Predisposition to dehydration might result from this.

It's imperative that you be well-hydrated at all times of the day. As the body loses more water, the risk of urinary tract infections and bladder discomfort increases.

Drink more water than the recommended daily amount of eight glasses. Other types of drinks can be added to the diet to help keep the body properly hydrated. You can also drink coffee and tea as part of your regular fluid intake. Ketosis is not greatly affected by coffee or tea alone, but it may be by the addition of additional substances. Select artificial sweeteners. Or, if you want, you may eliminate the sugar and have your coffee or tea with whole milk.

Fruit smoothies should be avoided in favour of protein shakes or power smoothies. Sugars in the fruits might cause ketosis to be disrupted.

While on a ketogenic diet, vegetable juices made from the authorised vegetable varieties are also a good option for a beverage.

INSTRUCTIONS FOR THE DIET

Begin by determining the proper daily calorie intake for each macronutrient (fats, carbs, and proteins).

Body Mass Index (BMI)

The following are methods for calculating body fat percentage:

For the ladies:

Percentage of Body Fat

Characteristic

(1 - 100 %)

5-9

• Usually, this isn't a viable option.

• All of the muscles are clearly visible.

• All muscles show signs of vascularity

• Extremely low levels of body fat

10-14

• The beach body look

• Arms and legs with limited vascularity

Some of the muscles appear to be separated from each other.

15-19

• A lean appearance

muscle separation is more difficult to see

Vascularity is reduced.

• Only the arms are vascularized.

20-24

• Men's typical range

muscles do not appear to be separated from one another

Very few striations or blood vessels are seen.

Abs are trim, yet they don't have a flabby look about them.

25-29

• Obese to the point of being considered overweight.

• Increase in the circumference of the waist

• Abdominal roundedness.

Small amount of subcutaneous fat at the nape of the neck

Muscles do not separate from one another.

• There is no vascularity to be seen.

30-34

• The abdomen seems more rounded.

• The hips appear to be smaller than the body and waist.

• The first signs of a chin adiposity

35-39

More than 40 inches in waist circumference

• The stomach grows larger and hangs down.

Over the age of 40

Obese in the extreme

• As more fat is stored, the abdomen and chest get larger.

deposited

• Difficult tasks to complete

For women, use the following:

Waist, breast, and thigh fat is more common in women than in men. Essential body fat in women is 8 percent, but it is just 2 percent in males.

Percentage of body fat (percent)

Characteristic

10-14

When it comes to bodybuilders, this is more common.

• Well-defined and clearly divided muscles

• All across the body, there is a noticeable vascularity. •

15-19

• Absence of body fat

• The hips, buttocks, and thighs are less defined.

Muscles that are clearly defined

• Arm and leg vascularity

Separation of muscle fibres

20-24

• The majority of female sports participants

Decreased visibility of muscle separation

• A physically fit body

The abdomen must be defined in some way

• A lack of definition in the arms and legs

25-29

The majority of women in this group are female.

neither too thin nor too fat

Hips with a swoop

• More fat in the buttocks and thighs.

30-34

Possessions begin to increase in size

• Fat accumulates around the hips, thighs, and buttocks. –

• The thighs and buttocks appear more rounded.

35-39

Facial and neck fat accumulates.

As the body begins to store fat, the stomach protrudes slightly.

• A waist measurement of more than 32 inches

40-44

• Fat builds in the thighs and hips and develops bigger.

• The average waist circumference is 35 inches.

Over the age of 45

Visible differences in hip and shoulder width

• A waistline of more than 35 inches is required

• The skin is dimpling.

Weight in terms of lean body mass

Acquire the weight of lean mass. This is a different weight from what is shown on the scale. Weight is multiplied by the percentage of body fat and then subtracted from the weight to get lean mass weight. The lean mass weight of a 120-pound individual with 25% body fat is 225 pounds. Calculate the total weight in pounds by multiplying 120 pounds by 0.25. (from 25 percent body fat). It's a total of thirty.

Add 30 pounds to the weight of 120 pounds to get the final weight. The lean body mass (90 pounds) is the effect of this exercise.

Calories in a Day

If you want to know how many calories you need to consume each day, multiply your total body weight by 15. The weight, in this case, is 120 pounds. Exponentiate by 15. (120 x 15). The end result is a calorie consumption of 1800 per day.

Reduce your daily calorie intake by 500 calories to kick-start fat burning. The fat burning process begins with just 1300 calories a day.

Weight reduction is the goal.

To lose a pound of fat in a week, cut your calorie consumption by 500 every week. Reducing the weekly caloric intake by 1000 calories will help you lose 2 pounds.

This figure shows how much of each macronutrient you should eat on a traditional ketogenic diet. There is a 5% carbohydrate restriction. 22.5 percent of the total daily calorie intake is made up of moderate protein, whereas 72.5 percent of the calorie intake is made up of fats. A person with epilepsy, for example, may consume as much as 90% of their daily caloric intake from fats.

Protein

A ketogenic diet necessitates moderate protein intake. The ketosis state might be disrupted if you eat a lot of protein. The similar cycle of carbohydrate metabolism occurs when the body converts excess proteins in the meal into glucose.

Muscle loss can occur as a result of insufficient protein consumption. When it comes to the growth and repair of the body's tissues, proteins are essential. Malnutrition and muscle atrophy can occur as a result of inadequate nutritional intake. In some cases, the harm may be irreparable.

A daily calorie intake multiplied by the ketogenic protein allocation yields your daily macronutrient consumption. The 20-25 percent protein proportion of a ketogenic diet may be obtained by multiplying the predicted daily calorie intake by 0.20 and 0.25. As a result, if you consume 1800 calories a day, your protein consumption will be between 360 and 450 calories. 4 calories are in per gramme of protein. As a result, a daily protein intake of 90 to 112.5 grammes is recommended.

Carbohydrates

Ten to twelve grammes of carbohydrates per kilogramme of lean body mass is advised. The unit of measurement for weight in the preceding example is pounds. Divide the lean mass weight by 2.2 (90 / 2.2) to arrive at the kilogramme equivalent. In kilos, the weight is 40.9, or approximately 41 kg.

If you increase this by ten (and again by 12), you'll have the daily carbohydrate consumption range.

In addition, the ketogenic diet recommends increasing the daily calorie consumption by 5% to 10%. The daily caloric consumption in this case is 1800. For a day's worth of carbohydrate intake:

1800 divided by a decimal of 0.05 is 90

One hundred and eighty

As a result, a 120-pound person on a ketogenic diet should consume no more than 90 to 180 calories per day in carbohydrates. In order to put your body into ketosis, the smallest dose is generally the most effective. Approximately 4 calories are found in each gramme of carbs.

A daily intake of 22.5 to 45 grammes of carbs is based on this calculation. These are the nett carbs, not the overall amount of carbs in a meal, that are being discussed.

Carbohydrate counting focuses on the nett carbohydrate intake. The overall carbohydrate content of a meal is calculated by subtracting the fibre content. Broccoli is a good example. Carbohydrates are 6 grammes in a cup. It has about 2 grammes of fibre per cup. By subtracting the fibre content from the total carb amount, you can determine how many nett carbs are in a serving of broccoli (6g-2g). The nett carbohydrate content is 4 grammes.

Weight reduction on the ketogenic diet can be achieved by limiting nett carbohydrates to an average of 20-30g per day. This, however, may be excessive. When making such a major change, it is important to proceed with caution.

Fats

After determining the protein and carbohydrate content, fats may be simply calculated. Basically, fat calories are calculated by subtracting the calories from carbs and proteins. There are 9 calories per gramme of fat.

For a calorie intake of 1800 per day, the formula is as follows:

carbohydrate-rich foods contribute between 90 and 180 calories per serving

360 to 450 calories from protein sources

Total daily calorie intake is equal to the amount of calories from fat consumed. - carbs - protein 1800 – 90 – 360 = 1350

1800-180 – 450 = 1170

For an 1800-calorie daily diet, the total amount of fat calories is between 1170-1350. There are 9 calories per gramme of fat. So,

More than 1170 calories divided by 9 is 130 grammes.

a calorie deficit of 9 grammes is equal to a calorie surplus of 1350 grammes.

If you're following a ketogenic diet and need to consume 1800 calories per day, your macronutrient breakdown is as follows:

Chapter Three

50 SIMPLE RECIPE IDEAS

Getting into ketosis is simple with these simple ketogenic meals.

Breakfast

In addition, there are "Power Eggs."

Three huge eggs

In a nutshell:

1 tablespoon of unsalted butter

In a separate dish, beat the eggs until they are light and fluffy. Amount of salt and pepper can be adjusted based on one's own preference.

Butter should be melted in a hot pan.

Eggs should be cooked to firmness.

Value as a Dietary Supplement:

caloric intake: 318

26.3 g of fat

1.8 grammes of carbohydrate are included in this serving.

17.4 g of protein

Fruity Power Pancakes

a single scoop of protein powder

14 cup of egg whites

2 tbsp. of almond milk

Two tablespoons of Greek yoghurt.

12 a medium-sized banana, mashed

34 cup of frozen raspberry

1 tbsp. ground cinnamon

Grind 1 tablespoon of chia seeds.

In a large bowl, combine all of the ingredients except the raspberries. Make a thorough stir.

Raise the raspberries to the surface. Mix it up a little bit and see if it's ready.

Applying a little mist of olive oil to a skillet over medium heat can help the dish come together faster.

Mixture should be poured into the pan. When the sides get brown, flip it over and cook the other side.

Continue to cook until the desired doneness is achieved.

Serve with plain Greek yoghurt.

Value as a Dietary Supplement:

A serving of this dish has 275 calories.

1g of fat

36 grammes of protein

There are 29 grammes of carbs in this dish

9g of fibre

Carbohydrate content: 20 grammes

Pudding made with chia seeds

3 tbsp. chia seed powder

1 cup of unsweetened skim milk

1 tbsp. cocoa butter

14 cup fresh or frozen raspberries

Sweetened condensed milk, 1/4 cup

Fork together the skim milk and chocolate powder.

Make sure to incorporate the chia seeds into the mixture.

For 5 minutes, let the mixture rest. Stir well and allow the mixture to rest for five minutes before serving.

Stir everything once more, then put it in the fridge for 30 minutes.

Serve with the raspberries on top.

Serves two people.

Per serving, there is a nutritional value of

235

Carbohydrates: 19g

Fiber: 8 grammes

There are 11 grammes of nett carbohydrates in this serving.

Fat content: 12g

30g of protein

• The Power Omelet is an excellent source of protein.

1 tbsp. of shredded spinach

plum tomato, one

1 Tablespoon of purple onion

Garlic

1 bundle of fresh basil

4-5 eggs' worth of whites

Egg whites, 2

2 Tablespoons of soy milk

Toss with a little salt and pepper if desired.

A good example of this is olive oil.

Egg yolk, egg white, and soy milk are all beaten together in a bowl. Salt & pepper to taste.

Slice up the tomato.

Trim and finely chop the basil leaves and the onions.

In a small frying pan, heat the olive oil over medium-high heat. Sauté the veggies for a few minutes over a medium heat. The veggies should be removed from the pan.

In the same pan, heat a small amount of olive oil before adding the eggs.

Take care not to overcook the eggs.

Cooked veggies should be spread over half of the eggs.

Fold the second part over the first.

Serve.

In terms of nutrition,

Nutritional information per serving: 203 calories

5 grammes of fat

20 grammes of protein

18 grammes of carbs

2 grammes of fibre

Carbohydrates, nett: 16g

• Muffins with cheese.

Two cups of almond flour.

14 teaspoon of salt

12 tsp. bicarbonate of soda

One cup of sour cream.

2 hens' eggs

1/8 cup of melted butter.

12 tsp of dried thyme

12 cup of shredded muenster

Shredded cheese or Colby jack, a cup of each

Set the temperature of the oven to 400 degrees Fahrenheit and prepare the dish.

Put cupcake papers in a muffin tin and bake as instructed.

Add all of the dry ingredients to a large bowl and mix thoroughly.

Beat the eggs in a separate basin.

Pour in the sour cream and butter.

Dry components are mixed with liquid. Add 1 tablespoon of heavy cream or water if the batter is too thick.

Add the cheese and mix it in until it's completely incorporated.

Fill muffin tins 3/4 full with batter and bake for 20 minutes.

Five minutes at 400 degrees should do it.

Reduce the oven temperature to 350 degrees Fahrenheit. Bake for a further 20 minutes, or until the tops are golden brown and crispy.

Remove from heat and top with butter before serving.

Amount of nutrients in each muffin

166

15 g of fat

g of protein

5 g of carbs

3 grammes of fibre

2 grammes of nett carbohydrates per muffin

• Butter-slathered Hard-Boiled Eggs

2 cooked whole eggs

1 spoonful of mascarpone cheese

a half-pound of butter

Toss with a little salt and pepper if desired.

Into a bowl, add the peeled and chopped hard-boiled eggs.

While the eggs are still hot, stir in the mascarpone cheese and butter until combined.

Make sure everything is well-combined. Salt and pepper to your liking.

Value as a Dietary Supplement:

42g of fat

A serving size of 14 grammes of protein.

There are 1g of carbs in this dish

-

Carbohydrates, nett: 1 g

430

Lunch/Dinner

• Stir-Fry.

Tablespoon Coconut Oil

A pound of ground beef

Approximately five medium-sized brown mushrooms.

A quarter of a medium-sized Spanish onion.

Two leaves of kale

12 cup of broccoli

A medium-sized red pepper, about half of it.

1 tablespoon of cayenne pepper

1 tablespoon of the Five Spices of China

Gather your ingredients and begin chopping.

Cut the mushrooms into thin slices.

A big skillet over medium-high heat should be used to cook the coconut.

After approximately a minute, add the onions.

Serve with the remaining veggies. 2 additional minutes of cooking time. Stir often to ensure even cooking.

Spices and ground beef should be added at this point. Cook for an additional 2 minutes.

Lower the temperature to medium-low.

Cook the meat, covered, until it's well-browned. This normally takes between 5 and 10 minutes.

Serve. This recipe yields three servings.

Per serving, there is a nutritional value of

Calories in single serving: 307

18 grammes of fat

7 g of carbs

29 g of protein

• Deviled Eggs with Butter

This recipe calls for 12 big hard-boiled and peeled eggs.

A quarter cup of finely chopped white onion

1teaspoon of black pepper

1 teaspoon of salt

Two teaspoons of melted butter

12 cup of mayonnaise

12 teaspoons of yellow mustard.

The eggs should be cut in half lengthways.

Place the white shells on a separate serving platter and set aside until ready to serve.

In a separate dish, separate the egg yolks from the whites.

With a fork, pulverise the yolks to a fine powder.

Add the other ingredients and stir thoroughly. Season to your preference.

The yolk mixture should be poured into the egg white shells.

Cover. Until you're ready to dine, keep the eggs in the fridge.

It yields 24 deviled eggs.

For one deviled egg, the nutritional value is:

81

Weight in grammes: 7 grammes of fat

g of protein

Carbohydrates: 0.5 g

Recipes for Ginger Beef

2 strips of 4-ounce sirloin

1 tablespoon of extra virgin olive oil

1 finely sliced onion

1 crushed clove of garlic

2 diced tomatoes, in a bowl

1/4 cup freshly grated ginger

Pour 4 tbsp. of apple cider vinegar

Toss with a little salt and pepper if desired.

Over medium-high heat, add oil to a large skillet. Place the steaks on the grill and cook them on both sides.

Toss in the garlic, onion, and tomato slices.

In a separate dish, combine the vinegar, salt, ginger, and pepper. Set aside in a bowl until ready to use. Make sure everything is well combined by giving it a good stir.

It's time to put the lid on the skillet. Turn down the heat a notch or two.

Simmer until all of the liquid is gone.

Serve.

Value as a Dietary Supplement:

There are around 208 calories in each serving.

Proteases: 31g

8g of fat

Carbohydrates: 3g

Meatloaf is a classic American dish.

Sausage that weighs 1lb

2 pounds of ground beef that is 85 percent beef

12 cup of Parmesan cheese in a dry grater

12 cup of almond meal

As much butter as you'd like.

5 minced garlic cloves

White onion, diced, 8 ounces (measure by weight)

1 cup peppers, chopped

Thyme leaves: 1 tbsp

1 tablespoon finely chopped fresh basil

14 cup freshly minced parsley

1/4 teaspoon black pepper ground

1 pinch of salt

Eggs, two, medium-sized

2 teaspoons of Dijon mustard

Sauce for Low-Carb Barbecue

14 cup heavy cream

An unflavoured gelatine teaspoon

Set the temperature of the oven to 350 degrees Fahrenheit and prepare the dish.

Spray butter into a 10-by-15-inch baking dish to grease it.

In a bowl, combine almond flour and Parmesan cheese. Set aside for now.

Cook pasta in a medium-sized pan on medium-high heat. Pepper and onion should be added to the butter. Sauté the vegetables for approximately 8 minutes, or until they're tender.

Set aside for cooling. Mince the veggies in a food processor until they are of a fine consistency.

In a separate bowl, combine the eggs, spices, pepper, salt, BBQ sauce, mustard, and cream. Mix the gelatine into this mixture and then add it. Wait for 5 minutes before serving. Add the minced onion mixture and stir well. Set aside after you've thoroughly combined the ingredients.

Make sure the steak and sausage are well combined. Mix for no longer than 5 minutes. The flesh will get harder as a result.

To this, add the egg and milk combination. Make sure everything is well-combined.

Toss in the almond flour and stir.

Stir until the mixture is no longer sticky and all the ingredients are well dispersed throughout. To make it less sticky, add a little extra shredded Parmesan.

Pour the mixture into a loaf pan, then shape it into a loaf. On all sides, leave an inch of space.

Cook meatloaf until it is browned and a meat thermometer inserted into the centre comes out at 160 degrees. This might take up to an hour. Let the beef loaf cool completely before slicing and serving.

This recipe yields 12 servings.

Each 5-ounce portion has the following nutritional value:

Calories in one serving: 409

33 grammes of fat

(23g) of protein

5-gram carbohydrate serving

1 g of fibre

Carbohydrates, nett: 4 grammes

Variations:

o In a food processor, mince 8 pieces of cooked bacon. Then add the egg mixture to the onion mixture and stir well.

Bake.

Value as a Dietary Supplement:

It contains 485 calories, 36 grammes of fat, 24 grammes of protein, 5 grammes of carbohydrates, 1 gramme of fibre and 4 grammes of nett carbohydrates. Bake.

Value as a Dietary Supplement:

Fat: 39 grammes, protein: 28 grammes, carbs: 6 grammes, fibre: 1 gramme, nett carbohydrate grammes

• Herb-Baked Salmon w/ Potatoes

12-pound chunks of salmon fillets

Tamari or soy sauce, about a half-cup

4 oz. of sesame oil

Ground ginger is around half a teaspoon.

Minced garlic: 1 teaspoon

1/2 tsp. basil, minced

Oregano leaves, about 1 teaspoon

Rosemary, half a teaspoon

The tarragon is 1/4 teaspoon.

Thyme is 1/4 teaspoon.

4 tablespoons of butter

Green onions sliced into half a cup

1 cup of finely chopped fresh shiitakes

Add the spices, tamari sauce, and sesame oil to a bowl and mix well.

Then seal the bag with the fish inside. Make sure to add the sauce.

With the skin side up, marinate for up to four hours in the fridge.

Set the oven to 350 degrees Fahrenheit.

Using foil, cover a baking dish.

In a single layer, place the fillets in the pan. Overlay the marinade using a spoon.

Bake the fillets for 10 to 15 minutes at 350°F.

Over medium heat, melt the butter.

Toss in the veggies to evenly distribute the dressing.

The fish should be taken out of the oven. Put a dollop of butter mixture on top of the salmon. The mixture should be applied to each fillet.

Bake for another 10 minutes at 350°F. Serve at once.

For an 8 ounce portion, the nutritional value is:

There are 353 calories in one serving.

Amounts of fat: 23 grammes

32g of protein

2 grammes of carbohydrate.

1g of fibre

1g of nett carbs

• Chicken with rosemary in a pan

6 ounces of skinless chicken breast

Butter is a tablespoon in size.

1 tsp. rosemary

a pinch of salt

Combine the salt and rosemary in a bowl. Then use it to coat the chicken with. Butter should be heated in a skillet over medium heat. Skin-side down first while roasting the bird.

Value as a Dietary Supplement:

480 calories are the recommended daily calorie intake.

0 grammes of carbs

Nutritional data: 35 grammes of protein

4.3 ounces

• Salmon Baked in the Oven

2 salmon fillets of 6 ounces

6 tbsp. of olive oil in a mild flavour

Mince two garlic cloves

Dried basil: 1 teaspoon per serving

Ground black pepper to a fine powder:

1 pinch of salt

Citrus flavouring: 1 tbsp

1 tbsp. chopped fresh parsley

Marinade: Combine the olive oil, parsley and basil with the garlic and lemon juice. Salt and pepper to taste, as well as the salt and pepper.

Preheat your oven to 350 degrees Fahrenheit. The marinade should be covered.

Refrigerate for at least an hour to allow the flavours to meld. Flip the fillets once in a while.

Set the oven to 375°F.

Seal the aluminium foil around the fillets with the marinade. Bake the salmon in a baking dish that has been sealed.

Bake for between 35 and 45 minutes, depending on the size of the dish.

Serving Size (for 6 ounces):

436

30 grammes of fat

37 grammes of protein

2 grammes of carbohydrates

1g of fibre

Carbohydrates, nett: 1 g

Soups

Soup with Zucchini and Carrots •

Two medium zucchinis, cut into tiny pieces, each serving.

1 medium onion

1 litre of chicken stock

Olive oil, 2 tsp.

1/2 cup coarsely chopped fresh dill

pepper, a tiny, one

Toss with a little salt and pepper if desired.

Warm up the olive oil. Salt & pepper to taste.

Add the chicken stock to the mixture. Season to taste with salt and pepper 10 minutes of simmering time.

Zucchini can be added at this point. When the zucchini is fork-tender, remove it from the heat.

The heat should be turned off at this point. The dill should be added.

Net Carbohydrate Value: 10g.

• Leafy Green Soup

Oregano, lovage, parsley, and sorrel leaves, 200 grammes each.

One litre of beef stock

The white part of an egg,

100 ml of creme fraîche

Clean up the leaves. When they're cut into long threads, they'll seem more like noodles than a pasta dish.

Prepare the beef stock by bringing it to a boil. Leaves can be added. Allow the mixture to simmer for a few seconds before removing it from the heat.

Five minutes cooling time is sufficient.

Serve yourself a few spoonfuls. For another minute, let it cool off.

The yolk and the crème fraîche should be mixed together in a cup.

Whisk the yolk and crème fraîche combination into the broth in a slow, steady stream to prevent the yolk from coagulating and making the soup grainy.

Put the broth and the leaves in a large saucepan and bring to a boil. Serve immediately after mixing.

Value as a Dietary Supplement:

Fatty Acids: 16.5 grammes

7.75g of protein

Carbohydrates: 7g

1.75 grammes of dietary fibre

Net Carbohydrates: 5.25g

Calories per kilogramme: 20

Salads

• A variety of salads

Mix 3 cups of salad greens together. Pour 2 tablespoons of salad dressing over the salad.

Glycemic Index (GI): 5

• Broccoli and cauliflower salad with steamed vegetables

Broccoli and cauliflower florets, each about a cup, should be combined. For best results, use a steamer. The cooking process will be halted as soon as the food is removed from the heat source. Taste and add salt and pepper or a spoonful of butter to your liking.

4g of nett carbs

Salad with a creamy dressing of greens

Mix a variety of lettuces together. Incorporate 4 cherry tomatoes. Add 3 ounces of your favourite cheese, grated or cubed. Just mix in the dressing and the cream. Combine all of the ingredients.

Carbohydrates removed from 1 gramme of body weight

In addition, there is a Keto Cobb Salad.

A cubed 100-gram portion of ham

2 pieces of turkey bacon

Two pieces of hard cooked eggs

4 slices of cherry tomatoes

2 cups of finely chopped Romaine lettuce

a diced half avocado

30 grammes of blue cheese

Cooking with extra virgin olive oil

For 3-4 minutes, cook the ham in a pan over medium heat.

Cut the hard-boiled eggs into pieces.

Layer the veggies in a serving dish.

Apply the dressing in a slick, even layer.

Value as a Dietary Supplement:

370

Fat content: 27g

7 grammes of carbs

46 g of proteins

• Egg salad a.k.a. egg salad

This recipe calls for 12 big hard-boiled and peeled eggs.

minced white onion, about a third of a cup

1 teaspoon of salt

1teaspoon of black pepper

12 cup of mayonnaise

Two teaspoons of melted butter

12 tsp of ground mustard

Cut the eggs into 14 inch chunks using a serrated knife.

Mix the egg with the rest of the ingredients well.

Keeping it in the fridge until you're ready to eat it is recommended.

This recipe yields roughly three cups.

Calories per serving (2 ounces):

Nutritional information per serving: 163 calories

Fat content: 14 g per serving.

g of protein

2 g of carbs

1 g of fibre

1g of nett carbs

Snacks

fried eggs with Gorgonzola cheese

Hard cooked and peeled six eggs

50 grammes of Gorgonzola cheese

100 ml of creme fraîche

1 tbsp. of spicy mustard

Fresh cilantro leaves

a spicy red pepper flakes

Remove the yolk by slicing the eggs in half and then slicing them in half again.

In a small bowl, combine the yolk and the rest of the ingredients.

Return the yolked mixture to the egg white halves and fold them in half. Serve chilled, at least two hours.

Value as a Dietary Supplement:

27 lbs. of extra body fat

15 grammes of protein

Carbohydrates: 2 grammes

Fiber content: 0.25 grammes

Nutritional Information Per Serving (g): 1.75g

Amount of calories in the body: 313

• Vanilla flavoured ricotta cheese.

Fat-free Ricotta cheese (2%), 200g

1 tbsp. fresh cream

There is one Vanilla Sachet in this Vanilla flavour.

Combine the ingredients in a large bowl.

Value as a Dietary Supplement:

Fat content: 18g

8g of protein

Carbohydrates: 3g

-

3 grammes of carbs are the nett carbs.

the following number of calories

Desserts

• Crispy, deep-fried snack of cheddar

Two 50-gram pieces of cheddar cheese

One teaspoon of almond flour

A single entire egg

One teaspoon of ground flaxseed

1 tbsp. hemp nut powder

1 tablespoon of extra virgin olive oil

Toss with a little salt and pepper if desired.

Over medium-high heat, place a frying pan. Add a tbsp. of extra virgin olive oil.

Add the salt and pepper to the beaten egg and whisk until smooth.

Combine the flaxseed meal, hemp nuts, and almond flour in a mixing bowl and stir well.

Spread the bread crumbs on the cheese pieces. Egg mixture first, followed by dry.

For each side, cook for 3 minutes. Serve warm.

Value as a Dietary Supplement:

Fat content: 48g

35g of protein

Carbohydrates: 5g

2g of fibre

3g of nett carbohydrate intake

588 kcal per pound

• Chocolate Creamy

Whey protein isolate, 25 grammes (1 scoop)

1 tsp. unsweetened dark cocoa powder (5g)

100 ml of 35% fat cream

1 tablespoon of sesame oil

5 drops of sweetener in the liquid

a teaspoon of psyllium husk

Protein powder, psyllium and chocolate should be mixed with 300ml of water. Ensure a good shake.

Toss in the sugar and sesame oil and mix. Mix thoroughly.

To avoid foaming, add the cream and combine, but do not shake.

Consume within 30 minutes.

Value as a Dietary Supplement:

Fat content: 52g

23g of protein

11 grammes of carbs

5 grammes of fibre

6g of nett carbohydrates

kilocalories: 591

Drinks

• Teas made from herbal ingredients

Boil some water and put in a spoonful of dry herbs, such as tea leaves, to brew. Drink through a strainer.

• A Raspberry Protein Smoothie.

Fresh 77g raspberries

Almond cream (1 cup)

PEANUT BUTTER, THE REAL DEAL (24g)

One-fourth teaspoon of cinnamon

14 tsp of ginger

In a blender, combine all of the ingredients. Serve.

Value as a Dietary Supplement:

There are 49 calories and zero fat grammes in 77 grammes of frozen raspberries; 11 grammes of carbohydrates and one gramme of protein.

29 kcal, 2g fat, 1g carbs, and 1g protein per cup of almond milk

Toasted nuts: 24g, 150kcal, 12fat5carbs6protein

• Smoothie with Espresso

1 cup of coffee, preferably espresso.

1 scoop of protein powder in the flavour vanilla

Five ice cubes

14 cup of Greek yoghurt

Cinnamon pinches

Stevia may be pried apart using a pin.

Blend all of the ingredients together until smooth.

Value as a Dietary Supplement:

Calories in per serving: 169

35g of protein

3 grammes of carbohydrates

1g of fat

Blend of coconut and coffee

1/2 cup unsweetened black coffee

2 heaping teaspoons unsweetened coconut flakes

1 tablespoon of coconut oil

Grinded flaxseed, about 2 teaspoons

Sweetener to taste in a liquid form

Flaxseed and coconut flakes should be well combined.

Add coconut oil to the mixture. Pour the hot coffee over the mixture and whisk it thoroughly.

Reduce the coffee's bitterness by adding 3-4 drops of liquid sweetener.

Value as a Dietary Supplement:

Fat content: 27g

Protein:4g

Carbs:7g

Fiber:5g

2 grammes of nett carbohydrates

kcal:277

• Beverages with a muddled flavour

• The Margarita

One-and-a-half tequila shots

1/4 tsp. orange flavouring extract

2 ounces of lime juice

Preparation of 1/4 cup of Crystal Light Lemon Lime

Ice that has been ground into fine powder.

Blend everything together until smooth. Mix until it becomes a slushy consistency. Lime slices are a nice garnish.

2 grammes of carbohydrate.

• Martini with Apples

Slice of apple

Vodka with 2 ounces of water

a shot of apple-flavored bourbon

Sugar syrup with a low glycemic index

Finely dice the apple slice. Stir well with a cocktail shaker.

Sweeten with the sugar syrup, if desired. ice and both kinds of vodka

Mix thoroughly. Pour into a martini glass and enjoy.

Carbohydrates: 2 grammes

cocktail with fresh blueberries and bourbon

Vodka with 2 ounces of water

Vodka flavoured with blueberries, 2 ounces

Blueberries, around 6 to 7, of a decent size

Sugar syrup with a low glycemic index

In a cocktail shaker, combine the blueberries and sugar syrup. Combine the two. Add ice to the mixture and then the two kinds of vodka. Mix thoroughly. Pour into a martini glass and enjoy.

Carbohydrates: 2 grammes

The Mojito.

1/2 cup sweetened condensed milk

7 to 8 Mint stems

1 tbsp. of low-carb sweetener

a single lime

Finely cut the mint leaves. Add low-carb sugar syrup to taste.

Segment and squeeze the lime juice into a glass after cutting it in half.

Pour in the rum, ice, and club soda, then adjust the flavour to your liking. Stir.

4 g of carbs

• Pina Colada slushie

3-ounce rum shot

2 cups ice cubes, crushed

A half-cup of sugar-free coconut milk or whipped cream

Pineapple syrup sugar-free

Blend all ingredients until smooth.

One drink is poured.

5 grammes of carbs per serving

Chapter Four

THE DIARY PROGRAM

Initiation to the keto diet is referred to as the 7-day low carb diet menu. The most severe carbohydrate restriction occurs at this period.

Here is an example 7-day eating plan for a low-carb ketogenic diet to get you started in ketosis.

Day One:

Breakfast consists of two scrambled eggs and a cup of coffee.

Salad with ham and grated cheese: 1 cup of mixed leafy greens (such lettuce, spinach, kale) Pork chops and veggies in a stir fry for dinner

Day two:

To start the day, make some eggs over easy.

Lunch consists of two sausages and a salad of mixed greens.

Savory Sirloin Steak with Kale Soup for Dinner

Day three:

Breakfast: An omelette with ham, vegetables, and cheese.

2-patty burger with Cobb salad for lunch

Dinner: Pork roast and cheesy baked broccoli

Day four:

Cream cheese rolls ups for breakfast.

Baked salmon with a green salad for lunch.

Steamed cauliflower with pan-grilled beef for dinner

Day five:

Pancakes with raspberries for breakfast.

Meatloaf with mixed greens for lunch.

Chili-pepper spare ribs and a green salad for dinner

On the sixth day,

Two deviled eggs and two sausages are included in this meal.

We had beef stir fry with greens for lunch.

Roasted chicken with skin on and roasted veggies in butter for dinner

On the seventh day,

Eggs Florentine for breakfast is a delicious option.

Grilled chicken wings with coleslaw for lunch

grilled salmon belly and mixed veggies for dinner, please.

Snacks

A ketogenic diet promotes frequent small meals and snacks. However, carbo-hydrate-heavy snacks are the norm for most people.

Sugar and starch are the main ingredients in most of them. Snacks may also be a source of confusion when it comes to the carbohydrate amount of the food. While the ketogenic diet might produce feelings of deprivation, eating may be a method to alleviate this. It's possible to overeat. Prepare the snacks in advance to avoid this. Label the containers and store them in the refrigerator. Make a note of the amount of carbs and calories they contain. Count them as part of your daily calorie and carb intake.

Snacking guidelines are provided below to help you get the most out of your snacking experience.

Nuts are a healthy and filling snack. Remember that they still include carbs, so ration them out.

Pig rinds are also a good choice for a snack. They are high in fat and might make you feel full.

• Cheese cubes: Sample a variety of cheeses by tearing them up into little cubes.

• Celery sticks dipped in peanut butter or cream cheese (vegetables with the lowest carbohydrate content).

There is no carbohydrate content in beef jerky, which makes it a terrific choice for a protein snack. Aside from the additions and fillers or the curing ingredient like sugar and honey, beef jerky may include hidden carbs. Pay close attention to the information on the packaging.

Cuts made with a sharp knife.

• Slices of pepperoni

• Wings of chicken

• Eggs that have been hard cooked

Bacon-wrapped sausages for serving as an appetiser

• Roll-ups; There should be an emphasis on meats and creams when it comes to fillings.

Chapter 9 teaches you how to decipher food packaging.

When including commercial or processed food into meals, it is simple to exceed the daily carbohydrate allowance. Carbohydrate-based fillers can be found in ready-made sauces and dressings, as well as pre-mixed spices. Carbo-hydrates are used in the manufacturing of batters and breadings. Carbohydrate fillers can be included in processed meats like sausages and bacon. Gluten, a carbohydrate, is commonly found in prepackaged meats.

The following names for sugar substitutes may appear on product labels and should be avoided:

High Blood Sugar (HbS)

There are two types of sorbitan:

"Sweetheart"

glucose dihydrochloride (glucodin)

Sucrose is a sugar.

Milk sugar is the primary source of lactose

It has a high amount of fructose

• Glucose • Maltodextrin

Maltose is a sugar derived from malt.

There are several types of maltodextrins.

• Yummy!

Truncation

Sweetener made from molasses

• Maple, corn, and golden syrup are all types of syrup.

Keep an eye out for these sugary ingredients that are not readily apparent.

Chapter 10: Reminders for a Successful Ketogenic Diet

Week one is a time for acclimatisation. During this period, discomforts and side effects are likely to worsen. There should be a progressive decrease in the negative effects when the adjustment phase is through.

• At initially, meal preparations may be a challenge. Set up a routine to make things easier and faster.

In the early weeks of a ketogenic diet, hunger pangs exacerbate the discomfort. Water laced with the artificial sweetener saccharine might help alleviate hunger pangs. Eating smaller meals more frequently might also help.

In order to save space, you should use smaller plates. As a result, the serving sizes are inflated. It also alleviates feelings of deprivation owing to the stringent dietary guidelines.

Steaming is the finest method for retaining the nutritional content of vegetables.

A broad variety of foods are still available to those who reduce their carbohydrate intake. The key is to think beyond the box.

Diets That Actually Work

Find a Diet that Works for You

Diets That Actually Work

When it comes to finding a diet that works, individuals who have struggled with weight or health concerns understand the difficulties. If a diet isn't working for you, try another one. The Mediterranean Diet and the Hypothyroid diet are two examples of diets that work well for most people. The Mediterranean diet is a way of life that many people in Europe follow, and it has been shown to improve their health and lifespan. For those with low thyroid hormone, the Hypothyroid Diet offers a list of foods that are beneficial for the body and those that are bad.

A diet that is successful for you should be followed religiously. In the end, dieting isn't a short-term strategy to lose weight or manage a medical problem. Rather, it's a long-term strategy that requires consistent effort. Dietary adjustments are part of a healthy lifestyle. Look at the diet as an initiation into an eating habit that you should sustain until your weight loss is complete or your thyroid condition is stabilised. Neither of these diets requires a lot of effort to follow. All of the ingredients for both are readily available, and both can be turned into delicious dishes with a little creativity.

The Mediterranean Diet is one of the world's oldest diets, and it has been shown to be effective in helping individuals maintain a healthy weight and general health, especially the heart, for thousands of years. In order to adhere to the Mediterranean Diet, one must eat foods that are naturally found in the area around the Mediterranean Sea. All kinds of fruits and vegetables, as well as the majority of meats and a substantial amount of seafood, are included. People in the Mediterranean area follow a diet they call the "Mediterranean way of life." This diet should be approached as a long-term lifestyle adjustment, not a short-term fad.

Our quality of life suffers when we are plagued with health problems that bring us pain, sickness, and other negative health situations. Our lives will improve if we are able to identify and address the underlying health conditions. In most cases, a healthy diet may be used to repair imbalances in our bodies and so improve our health. The recipes in this book are designed to aid those who have hypothyroidism, a disorder that affects the thyroid gland. With our diets, we can treat and conquer health difficulties, or at the at least, make us feel better.

One of the most common causes of low thyroid hormone production is hypothyroidism. Sluggishness is the end outcome when this happens to the metabolism. If it isn't treated, it can quickly spread throughout the body and become a full-blown disease. However, medication only addresses a portion of the problem. When it comes to addressing any health problem, including hypothyroidism, we need to look at our diets. This book is all about hypothyroidism diets.

The recipes in this book are all oriented at treating hypothyroidism or low thyroid hormone in the body. Ingredients that have been shown to help boost the immune system are used in each dish. A week's worth of meals may be planned with ease using the recipes provided. Before beginning any new diet, you should, of course, consult with your doctor. Verify that the meals you consume are compatible with the drugs you are taking. As before,

You may customise any recipe to fit your personal preferences and demands.

Every type of protein and taste is represented in the book's entrée section, which comprises 25 dishes. Try the Puerto Rican style tenderloin of pig or lamb if you're a meat lover. Turkey burgers, chicken with excellent mushroom sauce, chicken puttanesca, and a brandied beef tenderloin are all on the menu at the restaurant. These hypothyroidism-friendly meat dishes are guaranteed to be a success with the whole family, and each one provides a delightful option for those with hypothyroidism to eat healthy. Filling main dish dishes featuring Italian, Mexican, and Caribbean flavourings are included here.

Many diets leave you in the dark about what to serve as a side dish, which is unfortunate because side dishes are an important part of any meal.

There's no need for that in this book because the Hypothyroid Diet section has a wealth of side dish dishes.

The zucchini and sardine salad, the warm goat cheese salad, the seaweed salad, and the arugula and grilled chicken salad are all wonderful options. Sesame cucumber noodles, mashed sweet potatoes with chipotle, and a superb wild rice pilaff round out the menu.

With the hypothyroid diet, your breakfast may be anything you want it to be. In this collection of breakfast recipes, you'll find things like asparagus and sundried tomato frittata, raspberry and ricotta soufflé with blackberries, coconut-pumpkin pancakes, and eggs Benedict topped off with smoked salmon and artichokes. Egg Florentine wraps, a mushroom and cheddar omelette, morning quinoa porridge, and a flourless chocolate cake are all options. Some of the other breakfast recipes, like the chocolate cake and the coconut cheesecake bars, coffee custard, and the delicious coconut rum ice cream, may also be eaten as desserts later on.

The Mediterranean Diet and the Hypothyroid Diet can both benefit from the meal ideas in this book. As a first-time dieter with weight or thyroid difficulties, you should definitely give the diets a shot. You may start a healthy eating habit by following the Mediterranean diet and prioritising nutrition. You'll be able to attain your goal weight faster, feel better, and your immune system will build up to a healthy metabolism that will keep you feeling good as your body adjusts to the changes.

Chapter Five

GUIDELINES

Dietary Guidelines for the Mediterranean Region, Section 1

Any effective weight loss programme necessitates a greater focus on what you consume. However, even if you eat a healthy diet, you won't be healthy if you don't remember to plan your daily activities in a healthy way. Finding good information is essential if you're serious about your weight loss goals. There are several ways to use this knowledge to attain your aims.

You may want to go back in time for more natural and traditional diet-based health treatments if the excesses of current fringe diets are too much for your appetite.

More and more individuals are turning to the Mediterranean diet as a way to enhance their general health, whether they are trying to reduce weight or get rid of a chronic health issue.

If you're looking for an easy way to eat healthily while still enjoying your favourite foods, a Mediterranean diet may be just what you've been looking for.

In addition to being tasty, it's also excellent for you in many ways. Westerners first learned about the benefits of a Mediterranean diet in the middle of the twentieth century, when studies found that people in southern Europe, where many recipes are similar, had significantly longer life expectancies and were less likely to suffer from chronic diseases like heart disease and high blood pressure than their northern counterparts.

When it was heralded as the "veritable spring of longevity" based only on dietary considerations in early research, it may have been over-hyped a few decades ago. For example, most Southern Europeans were still working in agriculture at the time of the original research, and because private automobile ownership and public transportation were few (in the majority of places), the people walked almost everywhere they went. Early studies omitted to mention that an active lifestyle was part of the explanation to why Southern Europeans lived longer, healthier lives; as a result, the better work-life balance was overlooked.

It's a well-known fact that even the healthiest of diets won't do much good if you don't maintain an active lifestyle.

While human involvement played a key effect in which crops became dominant, the foodstuffs that make up the Mediterranean diet were based more on the region's early inhabitants' practical understanding than on any profound old wisdom.

There was a far greater variety and plenty of food in the Mediterranean than in places with less favourable climates, such as those with short growing seasons and a need for food to endure through the long winters. People in the Mediterranean ate a far broader range of foods than those in the north, who relied mostly on bread, preserved meats, and a little amount of cheese.

The Mediterranean diet is a seafood-heavy one, just like the sea that bears its name. The winding coasts and cliffs

Most southern Europeans had access to fresh fish, clams and mussels, whereas most northerners had only tasted salted cod that had been marinated for six weeks on the back of a mule in the summers on its trip interior from the Atlantic Ocean. So, is it really a shock that the majority of Germans have developed a taste for sausage?

There was always a supply of fresh vegetables available in the local markets, so residents never had to resort on rat-infested grain stores like their neighbours in the sub-arctic.

Trade and the passage of time also played a role. The Mediterranean was a common route for the peoples who lived along its perimeter even before the Romans arrived. It was through these early trading networks that the olive, citrous, and grapefruits, as well as chickpea and other legumes, which comprise the heart of Mediterranean diet, were distributed and then mass-produced on the vast Roman villas that dotted the body of water they, not unjustifiably, dubbed Mare Nostrum, or "Our Sea".

It was principally exported cash products like grapes and wool while inexpensive and simple to grow cereals were made accessible for the army of agricultural labourers and slaves that supported it. For the Romans, it was obvious that they needed to feed their enormous workforce in the most cost-effective manner possible. Due in large part to the Roman Empire's 1000-year period of political and economic unification, many of the components that make up today's Mediterranean diet were consumed across the whole area thousands of years ago.

Over 30% of calories come from fat in the average Mediterranean diet. But the artery-clogging saturated fats found in red meat and other animal fats make up just 8% of the total fat intake. This is largely because red meat is eaten so rarely and olive oil is prefered as a cooking medium. Geopolitical factors come into play yet again here. Dairy was the primary use of animals in the Mediterranean because of the densely packed farms between mountains and deserts. Lamb was the only red meat consumed in Southern European diets before to the introduction of modern eating habits, and even then only sparingly, as wool was the primary source of clothing.

This isn't a normal Mediterranean diet, by any stretch. To cook with lard and butter in Northern Italy, for example, olive oil is solely used to flavour salads and vegetables.

Most people in North Africa abstain from drinking wine.

When it comes to your health, restricting your meal's ingredients to those usually found along the Mediterranean will bring long-term advantages and a depth of taste that is rarely seen in the "fat-reduction" diets touted by one weight loss expert or another.

Basic Components & Preparation Instructions

"Garbage in, garbage out," as computer programmers like to say about code, applies to the materials we use in our meals. To get the benefits of a Mediterranean diet, the first step is to familiarise yourself with its components and incorporate them into your regular diet.

Chapter Six

FOODIES

When cooked and processed to the bare minimum, vegetables retain the majority of their antioxidants, which are essential for good health and long life. Even more importantly, the wide range of vegetables and fruits that are regularly consumed allows those who struggle with diets a better chance of succeeding because of the wider options accessible.

Some of the most important Mediterranean fruits and vegetables are citrous fruits like oranges, grapefruits, and lemons.

Artichokes

Artichokes are actually the blossom buds of a species of thistle plant, which have been prized for their taste since ancient times. Because just a little portion of each blossom is edible, it's not a good idea to consume artichokes uncooked. In fact, even seasoned chefs have a difficult time preparing raw artichokes. Cooked, the soft bottoms of the buds and the centre of the plant are referred to as the "heart" of the artichoke.

savour every mouthful. If you buy raw artichokes, avoid ones with leaves that point out from the plant's centre, as they'll be primarily inedible fibre and hence more expensive to prepare. Artichokes should be baked in butter for a typical artichoke preparation. When the artichokes are done, drizzle them with a little olive oil and vinegar and serve them up. Alternatively, pre-cooked artichokes can be used for a fast snack. Most stores carry them in cans and jars.

Figs

The fig, a sweet fruit from the Ficus carica tree, is a popular delicacy in the Mediterranean region (fig tree). This tree is native to the Middle East, but thrives in Mediterranean climates because to its ability to adapt. Figs are rich in antioxidants, flavonoids, and polyphenols, and are a good source of fibre. Because of their high fibre and calcium content, they're an excellent food for building and maintaining healthy bones in children and adults alike.

The shelf life of fresh figs is extremely short. If you're looking for dried or preserved figs, you'll have a better chance of finding them. If you can get your hands on some fresh figs, try dipping them in honey or sprinkling some chocolate on them for a truly decadent treat.

Eggplants

Aubergine is the common name for Eggplant in Europe. Cooked in savoury recipes, it is commonly consumed.

Fruits and vegetables are both incorrectly labelled as "vegetables" when they are actually fruits.

Mediterranean cuisine is well-known for its use of eggplant. For Baba Ganouj, Lebanese and Israelis grill eggplant before combining it with tahini, lemon juice, minced garlic, salt, and other flavours. It is served with a warm pita bread. A essential element in Ratatouille, a Southern French vegetable relish with tomato, garlic, zucchini, onion and herbs Eating Moussaka, a traditional Greek dish, would be impossible if eggplant weren't included.

The bitter fluids in most Mediterranean eggplants must be drained before cooking.

Salting slices of eggplant and letting them sit for a time is the best way to achieve this. The fluids will be drained out, and the meat will be succulent.

Beans and legumes are also included in this category.

In contrast to many of the Mediterranean diet's beans and legumes, which arrived from Europe in the 15th century, some have been around for millennia. In Spanish cooking, both black and red beans are common ingredients. Beans like as fava, kidney, and lima are also often used in regional cuisine. Throughout the Western Mediterranean, such dishes as Spanish garbanzo soup rely heavily on chickpeas, while in the eastern Mediterranean, tahini and chickpeas are combined to make a delectable humus, a staple food especially popular in areas like the eastern Mediterranean and the North African coast.

Leafy greens can be used to make a salad with a Mediterranean flair. This salad is a great way to get a wide variety of fresh vegetables into your diet. Regularly consume roasted vegetables such as peppers and eggplant. Strike meat from your diet two days a week for optimal health advantages. Protein isn't the only thing you can get from eating meat. Beans and lentils are excellent sources of high-quality protein.

Foods derived from aquatic life

It is common for American grocery shops to have small fish counters and huge meat counters. A lot of red meat and very little seafood are staples of the typical American diet.

Increase your consumption of seafood and fish. They have a low calorie count and a high concentration of omega-3s.

There is a long history of seafood in the diets of people in the southern European region, dating back to Julius Caesar's time. Southern Europeans, by and large, reside within a radius of 20 miles.

miles and miles of ocean. As a result, they have easy access to meals high in iron. Northerners, on the other hand, live off the land and consume a lot more red meat as a result. Because fish could not be transported very far without deteriorating, this was made possible by straightforward logistics.

To preserve the nutrients in your seafood, cook it in one of four ways: sautéed, grilled, steamed, or roast it. Is deep-frying in fat a bad idea?

Mixing calamari with pasta or rice is an example of a healthy alternative to frying. You

It's possible to produce a Spanish Paella by adding calamari, rice, mussels, and red peppers.

Olive Oil

Staying clear of saturated fats and hydrogenated oils should be a clear indicator. These two health robbers have no place in a healthy Mediterranean diet. Some of the fat in the Mediterranean Diet comes from fish and cheese, but olive oil makes up the lion's share of it. There is a lot of demand for olive oil in the Mediterranean area. Olive trees thrive in an area where grazing space is in short supply. Several litres of oil may be produced from each tree each season. Olive oil is an excellent salad dressing, butter substitute for bread, and nutritious food in general. Olive oil has been shown to reduce LDL (bad cholesterol) levels and is a rich source of antioxidants, according to research. In both cases, cardiovascular disease can be prevented.

5. Herbs such as basil, oregano, and garlic

garlic, which has several health advantages, is a common ingredient in Mediterranean cuisine.

Garlic has a number of health advantages, including:

Contains a high concentration of anti-inflammatory and immune-boosting antioxidants.

Has the anti-cancer agent germanium in it. More germanium is found in garlic than in any other herb.

Anti-inflammatory properties lower blood pressure, serum triglycerides, and LDL-cholesterol, and prevent arteriosclerosis, which lowers the incidence of heart attacks and strokes,

Enhances the health of joints. Garlic eaters were shown to have a lower risk of osteoarthritis, according to research.

Infusing garlic into your cooking oils or adding some to your pasta water is an easy way to boost your intake of garlic.

Spices like basil and oregano can be used to enhance the flavour of a dish. You won't have to worry about upping your salt intake by flavouring your food instead.

It contains acetate, bisabolene, carvacrol, caryophylllene and other compounds that have both internal and external health advantages. The oils and leaves of basil and oregano are both sources of these compounds, making them both sources of both internal and external benefits.

Magnesium, which is abundant in basil, helps blood flow more freely by relaxing blood arteries.

Eating basil on a daily basis has proven to be beneficial for many people. Antibacterial properties have been found in basil, according to research. Both parasites in the intestines and bacteria resistant to modern antibiotics are defeated by these ingredients.

For stomach issues such as indigestion, cramps, and constipation, use basil oil. Colds, flu, and sinus infections can all be helped with this remedy. Asthma and bronchitis have been shown to benefit from its use.

Basil's numerous health benefits make it a wise choice to keep some on hand at all times. Simply said, there is no reason why you can't plant this easy-to-grow herb. Your kitchen should have plenty of sunlight and a large enough pot to support healthy root growth.

Pesto sauce, which features basil as the key component, makes it simple to incorporate into your diet. For Pesto sauce is a delectable accompaniment to any meal.

Boil 2 cups of spinach and 1 cup of basil together, then add some crushed pine nuts, olive oil, and salt to taste.

It's also possible to sprinkle a few basil leaves on top of your favourite dish.

Basil oil, which has antibacterial components, may be added to your salad dressing to make your veggies safer to consume.

Herbs, both dried and fresh, enhance flavour while also providing several health advantages.

6. Unrefined Foods

Bread, rice, and pasta come to mind when one thinks of the Mediterranean. Bread seasoned with cheese and olive oil is a go-to lunchtime snack. Throughout the Eastern Mediterranean region, flatbreads and pita are the most common form of bread. All of the nutritional benefits of wholegrain versions of these unleavened breads can be found in a small package.

To lose weight on the Mediterranean diet, you should stick to whole grain carbohydrate sources. A little Baba Ghanouj, Hummus, or olive oil can liven things up a touch.

Most Italians love pasta, but it can be included in a Mediterranean diet as long as you avoid the hearty northern Italian recipes that were developed to help people survive the bitterly cold winters in northern Italy, with their heavy cream sauces, thick cheese lathering, and use of fatty sausage or meatballs. With some shellfish like mussels or clams and a little garlic and olive oil or pesto sauce, pasta is often served simple in the south.

In addition, bear in mind that the health benefits of Southern Europeans are mostly due to a more laid-back and socially-minded society. When it comes to lunch in the United States, for example, most people have just 30 minutes to eat, move, and get back on their feet. Often, I'm the only one around. Anyone seen partaking of an alcoholic drink in broad daylight may be frowned upon, even sneered at publicly, doing so in front of work colleges may even result in a long-winded speech from the boss. Southern Europeans will typically enjoy long lunch breaks, typically about 2 hours (In Spain, its followed by the siesta, during which the entire country essentially closes for business) with workmates, family or friends with a full bottle or two of drink lubricating the conversation. People enjoy life rather than just survive it, therefore they don't eat for the sole purpose of fueling their bodies; they eat because they want to!

Yogurt and Cheese

Dairy products were traditionally produced because cows were too expensive to raise for human use on a regular basis. Traditionally, yoghurt was the most popular because it was simple to make and kept longer without refrigeration than fresh milk, which was especially useful during the hot summer months. The plain variety, with fresh fruits or honey as a flavouring, was a common Roman breakfast dish.

In comparison to their northern counterparts, many feta and Brie cheeses from the Mediterranean region are softer and less aged. This is because Southern Europeans didn't have as much of a need for long-lasting food sources due to the absence of a long, snowy winter. In the next section, we'll explain why cheese and yoghurt are so vital to our diets.

Sources of Protein

In order to maintain a healthy diet, it is essential to consume adequate amounts of protein. Each serving of Mediterranean cheeses such as feta, mozzarella, and goat cheese contains a significant amount of protein, making them all similar. Keeping in mind that protein is essential to muscle tissue growth is essential. The more muscle you have, the faster your metabolism will run, resulting in a greater rate of weight loss. Another great source of low-fat protein is the seafood, beans, and legumes discussed in the previous chapter. Poultry, chicken, and lamb are commonly eaten, but only in moderation, usually three times each week. Rich foods often incorporate chicken, for example.

Vitamins C and M

Yogurt and cheese are staples in the diets of those living along the Mediterranean coast. Calcium and magnesium may be found in abundance in each of these meals. You need calcium and magnesium not just for strong bones, but also for proper communication between your brain and body. Your body's ability to absorb nutrients like omega-3 fatty acids and unsaturated fats contained in olive oil is boosted by a diet high in protein and healthy fats. The minerals included in cheese are more effective when a Mediterranean diet adherent consumes a balanced amount of protein and fat.

Low Saturated Fats and "Good" Cholesterol Foods

Cholesterol is a necessary component of the human body, despite the fact that excessive amounts are hazardous. It regulates the movement of water and a slew of other vital chemicals throughout your body. In order to produce hormones like oestrogen and testosterone, your body needs cholesterol. To correctly digest high-fat diets and adequately process vitamins A, D, and E, your liver needs a sufficient amount of bile acid bilirubin. Good cholesterol levels can be increased while "bad cholesterol levels" can be kept within acceptable ranges by including some of the low-fat cheeses popular in the Mediterranean diet. Cheese prepared from goat and sheep's milk is prefered by many residents of the Mediterranean coast. The monounsaturated fats included in goat and sheep cheese contribute to a healthy cardiovascular system.

Contains a plethora of B Vitamins

Everybody is aware of the importance of vitamins, but those listed in the B-complex category are even more crucial to overall health. Vitamins B-6, B-12, and niacin are found in abundance in the Mediterranean diet's constituents. These vitamins act as catalysts for the conversion of the numerous proteins, lipids, and carbohydrates found in your stomach into effective fuel for muscular growth and energy generation. In the Mediterranean diet, high amounts of b vitamins may be found in foods like chickpeas and lentils and whole grains and seafood.

Healthy Eating Patterns Found in the Mediterranean

While their industrialised, fast expanding northern neighbours have regarded the Mediterranean shoreline a traditional, economically backwards region for the previous few hundred years, modernity has finally arrived in these nations. Even while urban residents have adopted certain contemporary habits, such as driving and watching TV for lengthy periods of time, rural residents continue to live in a way that naturally encourages long and healthy lives, in addition to their good food. Economic and cultural considerations both have a role in this.

Get Some Sleep, the First Healthy Mediterranean Habit

Agriculture is still a major source of employment for many Southern Europeans. The same family may have owned and operated a farm or vineyard for a dozen generations or more. There is no five-month winter break in the Mediterranean climate since most locations can grow diverse crops year-round because of the warm, rainy winters and hot, dry summers, unlike their northern neighbours. The fact that they spend so much time outdoors implies that they make a lot of vitamin D through increased levels of skin vitamin D production.

People in sunny areas with similar conditions, such as New Zealand, have lower incidences of skin cancer than those in southern Europe. One explanation is the increased pollution levels in upper atmosphere, which block some UV rays; another is that people living around the Mediterranean coast have developed a genetic tolerance for sunshine over thousands of years.

There is no doubt that spending a lot of time outside, allowing your body to manufacture its own vitamin D, is good for your health.

Walking is one of the best ways to maintain a healthy Mediterranean diet and lifestyle.

Due to the fact that many of the cities and villages in southern Europe date back to the Middle Ages, they are particularly pedestrian-friendly. When it comes to daily commuting vs. driving, European Mediterranean inhabitants walk far more frequently than their American counterparts. It's not just that Mediterranean towns and villages tend to be more compact; the town square, also known as the agora (Greek), the forum (Roman), the plaza (Spanish), and the piazza (Italian), has long been the centre of social life in these communities. It's also where local cafes, churches, government offices, and open-air markets can be found. Today, young couples, families, and retirees congregate in these historic locales on any given evening to celebrate life.

Health and Happiness Go Hand in Hand in the Mediterranean

On the Mediterranean culture, social connections are viewed as more significant than their economic status. When it comes to happiness, Southern Europeans tend to focus more on the quality of their social and familial relationships than do their Anglo-Saxon counterparts.

Not only does this apply to rural areas, but the whole population is practically linked to one other. On the Mediterranean, returning from vacation is more usual than in other parts of the world where returning home and catching up on one's job is acceptable.

a split in time (except, of course, in a family farm or business).

People tend to "get along" better with each other outside of the context of family life. A frequent pastime in the region is playing a game of dominoes or lawn bowling with folks you've just met in the cafés and squares.

Southern Europeans appear to have a decreased incidence of worry, stress, depression, heart disease, and depression as a result of increased time spent with loved ones and friends engaged in social and cultural hobbies.

A "Mediterranean Mindset" is a useful complement to taking use of the food of the Mediterranean, regardless of whether or not you work on a farm or whether getting around town requires a car.

In addition to keeping you physically healthy, spending more time with your family will have a profound effect on your personal well-being.

Benefits for Health

In comparison to the Western diet, there is little in common with the Mediterranean diet food pyramid. To put it simply, red meat is at the top of the pyramid and is eaten just a few times a month. A few times a week, eggs, chicken, and fish are offered. Yogurt and cheese in little amounts are routinely ingested. Every meal includes olives and olive oil as a common side dish. Fruits and vegetables, as well as nuts and legumes, form the foundation of the Mediterranean diet. The bottom of the food pyramid is made up of pasta, bread, and other grains. Cardiovascular disease and high cholesterol can be reduced by following the Mediterranean diet. Olive oil and cheese, which are high in good fats, are partly to blame, as is a more contented cultural attitude that places a higher value on spending time with family and friends than on earning a living.

Several diets have been identified, but the Mediterranean diet has the strongest evidence of health benefits, including a reduction in mortality.

The Mediterranean diet's high consumption of dietary fibre and substitution of unhealthy saturated fats with beneficial monounsaturated fats have earned it widespread acclaim.

Westerners have a long history of aversion to salt, so the high salt level of the Mediterranean diet comes as a surprise. In the Mediterranean diet, olive oil-based salad dressing is a common ingredient, as are olives, anchovies, and capers. In light of this fact, consider that our bodies rely on salt and require a lot of it each day. According to research, Southern Europeans do not experience the same levels of cardiovascular disease as the rest of the West. Because they eat less red meat, Southern Europeans aren't exposed to as much saturated fats as Westerners.

If you decide to go from a Western diet to a Mediterranean one, you'll want to reduce your salt intake until your body adjusts to the new food regimen.

Of course, the Mediterranean diet isn't the only way to get the health advantages of this lifestyle. Complete the image with a healthy diet, regular physical activity, and outside work.

The higher life spans of the inhabitants of Southern Europe can be attributed to genetics, but it is a minor factor.

The risk of heart disease was shown to be considerably higher among Mediterranean inhabitants who adopted the less active and fat-laden diet of Westerners.

People who eat traditional meals have a significantly lower risk of heart disease than those who don't.

The disparity between the geographic incidence of heart disease and the Mediterranean diet's overall advantages for excellent heart health is mostly associative in nature.

Research in the field of medicine

However, while it was well-known that Mediterranean people lived longer and better lives, little effort had been put into proving this until the mid-20th century. First, a study found that Crete's male residents had an extremely low risk of heart attacks, despite the fact that they consumed a lot of fat. Olive oil, bread, fresh fruit and vegetables, fish, and fresh dairy products are all staples of the Mediterranean diet in this area.

Taking the low mortality rate as a given, the Lyon Diet Heart Study set out to demonstrate that anyone following a diet comparable to that observed in the Cretan region might reap the same advantages. Vitamin C-rich fruits and wholegrain breads were also a component of the new diet, as was a significant reduction in red meat. Over the course of the study's several years, the death rate of participants from all causes was significantly lowered by 70%! The supervisory committee opted to end the trial early because of these results, which were deemed so remarkable that the study could be made public immediately.

The results of this study inspired other research teams to investigate the potential health benefits of a Mediterranean-style diet beyond heart health. Traditional Mediterranean diets have been linked to lower risk of type 2 diabetes, according to a study published in 2008. More than 13,000 college-aged students, all of whom did not have diabetes at the time of the study, had their eating habits monitored for a decade.

After the ten-year study concluded, some of the participants were still being tracked by the researchers. Additionally, it was shown that people who continued to eat a Mediterranean-style diet had a diabetes risk that was 80% lower.

Health researchers from the UK Medical Institute found that people who consume elements common to the Mediterranean diet in their diet are less likely to suffer from cancer and heart disease, according to a more detailed medical study published in 2008. Overall mortality was reduced by 9%, cardiovascular mortality was reduced by 9%, and cancer mortality was reduced by 6%, according to the findings. A 13 percent lower risk of getting Parkinson's and Alzheimer's disease was also found, according to the study.

There is evidence to suggest that specific parts of the Mediterranean diet are more directly responsible for the general reduced mortality risk than other items like grains, dairy, and seafood. This is based on a research published in the same Journal in 2009.

Moderate alcohol use, as well as a diet rich in fruits and nuts, are all linked to a decreased risk of premature mortality. Mitterrand components can help keep the brain healthy by lowering the number of micro strokes that play a significant role in senility, according to a study published in February 2010.

Consequently, there is an abundance of scientific data confirming the usefulness of the in addition to tasting excellent, presenting a wide variety of delectable components, and encouraging well-being.

Numerous studies have shown that following a Mediterranean diet lowers the chance of developing a variety of chronic illnesses. Because of this, the Mediterranean Diet's effectiveness as a translational paradigm for encouraging better living should come as no surprise.

Supplemental Dieting and Health Advice

A pet may be a great workout buddy if you're following a Mediterranean diet and working out with it. Having a pet as a weight-loss motivator and supporter is a unique experience. There are several ways to exercise with your pet. You and your friend will have a great time, but you'll also be helping yourself shed pounds.

Fruits are a healthier alternative to sugary munchies. The fibre, vitamins, and minerals included in fruits make them a better alternative for snacking than candy bars, chocolates, and other junk food, as well as satisfying Mediterranean snacks like hummous and pita bread.

If you want to improve your health, make friends with people who are physically active and healthy. You may use these folks as role models to help you reach your weight loss objectives. Additionally, you may be able to learn new strategies for slimming down.

Ensure that you drink enough of water throughout the day to keep your body hydrated. It is possible to shed water weight if you drink half a gallon of water a day and eat less for a week. In order to maintain a healthy weight reduction, avoid these methods and boost your total diet and exercise level.

Look for healthful options along the store's perimeter. In the next section you'll find a list of foods to consume from all four food groups. Center aisle goods tend to be pre-packaged, preservative, salt, and sugar-laden, and often lack the necessary components needed for a healthy diet. This is a little-known grocery store fact. Avoiding these aisles will decrease your likelihood of making a purchase.

Keep a daily eating and activity journal to keep tabs on your progress. People who maintain a record of their eating and exercise habits are more likely to notice trends and so be more successful in their weight loss efforts. Some people lose a significant amount of weight just by paying closer attention.

Sucking on some ice when you're craving a snack or a piece of junk food is a terrific technique to keep yourself from overindulging. An need to eat can be satiated by sucking on an ice cube.

To lose weight, you must understand the significance of following a healthy diet. Get rid of all the things in your kitchen that aren't going to help you lose weight and replace them with Mediterranean staples. The first step in losing weight is to eat more of these nutritious meals.

When you're trying to lose weight, avoid wearing a lot of loose clothing. Loose clothing is a frequent way for overweight persons to hide their size. You shouldn't worry about hiding your figure; instead, wear whatever makes you feel good. The more form-fitting your apparel, the more likely it is to make you aware of how much you weigh.

Don't be late for bed every night. A minimum of eight hours of uninterrupted sleep per night is recommended for

adults. Staying up late doesn't help you lose weight, as common belief would have you believe. You'll have a healthy metabolism if you get enough sleep.

Weight gain is inevitable if you eat without paying attention to portion sizes. Your weight reduction attempts will suffer if you aren't aware of what you're putting in your mouth at all times, which might lead to overeating. Eat less if you're conscious of how much you're taking in at each meal.

You can keep up your weight loss plan by eating leftovers. Prepare enough leftovers for the next day's lunch from your nutritious evening meal. For the entire week, you can make even more. This also makes it easier to put together a quick and easy supper the next day.

Many times hunger symptoms are mistaken for boredom or thirst. Wait 15 minutes before you succumb to a need. Drink water and go for a stroll for 15 minutes. Eat something if you're still feeling hungry.

French fries are a universal favourite. Every weight-loss plan has been derailed by them. The Mediterranean diet does not include a lot of potatoes, but when they do, they are usually boiled or baked rather than deep-fried.

Instead of packing on the pounds, consider baking your French-fries if giving them up isn't an option. Cut the potato into fries and coat them with olive oil before frying. Add salt and pepper and rosemary to the slices before roasting for 30 minutes at 400 degrees. Bake for a further 10 minutes after loosening with a spatula. You won't miss the deep-fried ones because they taste fantastic with ketchup and have a reduced fat level.

If you want to lose weight, you must avoid foods that make you crave more. The fact that you're in charge of your environment helps a lot. Trigger foods should not be brought into your house, automobile, or place of employment.

Consumption may occur even if you aren't hungry if you are frequently exposed to certain foods.

Instead of having your biggest meal of the day at night, eat it during midday. If you often have a sandwich for lunch, consider switching it up to supper. It makes lot more sense to eat more during the day and less at night since you burn far more calories during the day than you do at night.

Keep a healthy weight and you'll have a long and happy life ahead of you. If you want to achieve in the long run, you have to change the way you live each and every day. Make the changes you want to see in your life and your body with the resources you have at your disposal. Count on your own abilities!

The Hypothyroidism Diet, Section 2

Hypothyroidism is a condition in which the thyroid gland is underactive.

It is hypothyroidism, a disorder that occurs when the thyroid gland is unable to generate enough thyroid hormone to maintain a healthy metabolism. Thyroid hormone is one of the most critical hormones involved in the way that the human body consumes energy from the food that we eat and as such, hypothyroidism has an influence on practically every system and every organ in the body. More than 5% of adolescents and adults in the United States are affected by hypothyroidism, a disease in which the thyroid gland produces inadequate amounts of hormone.

One of the most common causes of thyroiditis is inflammation, which can be caused by a variety of reasons such as genetics, exposure to radiation for cancer, Hashimoto's disease, and pharmaceutical side effects. Symptoms of hypothyroidism include weight gain, a lack of energy and dry skin, as well as sadness and sensitivity to cold.

However, hypothyroidism sufferers have a brighter future ahead of them. Even while many people may successfully control their illness with diet and exercise rather than relying on drugs, these treatments are becoming more and more popular.

People with hypothyroidism are still debating what foods they can and cannot take, but a healthy, well-balanced diet that offers the required vitamins, minerals, and other nutrients is the ideal diet for hypothyroidism sufferers.

The Cookbooks

For this cookbook, we've avoided cruciferous vegetables like broccoli and cauliflower, which many nutritionists believe might worsen thyroid issues, in favour of other meals. Although many individuals with hypothyroidism cannot take them in large doses, if you can't bear to live without them, you could choose to add them in moderation.

Nutritional-balanced dishes that support endocrine health, particularly thyroid function, are the focus of this book's recipes. Even more significant is the fact that you'll find a wide selection of recipes here. You don't have to stick to a strict diet just because you have hypothyroidism; there are plenty of foods you may eat that are safe for you.

When it comes to cooking, there is no limit to what you may create. With the recipes in this book as your guide, you'll soon find yourself mastering the art of cooking and developing your own personal favourites. You can play around with the quantities of the spices and other ingredients in these recipes to find the right balance for your palate.

Speak to your doctor before beginning any new diet to get their opinion.

As a result of your hypothyroidism, your doctor may prescribe that you consume certain foods or take certain supplements to assist manage your condition, depending on the origin and severity of your hypothyroidism.

Once you've gotten the go-ahead from your doctor, you may start experimenting with these dishes to see how much creativity you can still bring to the kitchen while still managing your hypothyroidism with the proper nutrients.

When feasible, organic products should be used whenever possible, even if they aren't explicitly included in these recipes. It's better for you in general, and it's also good for managing hypothyroidism.

Entrées

Caribbean Style Grilled Pork Tenderloin (Or Lamb)

The serving size is 8 people.

Ingredients:

2 pounds of trimmed pig (or lamb) tenderloin

Crushed garlic from six to eight cloves, chopped or minced, in a garlic press

2 tbsp thinly chopped green onions

More than a half-dozen fresh limes

1/3 cup chopped fresh cilantro

dried oregano, 3 tbsp

3 tbsp. of black pepper.

1 tsp of salt per serving

1-2 tablespoons cumin seed

oil, olive, 2 tbsp (use extra virgin olive oil if possible)

Preparation:

In a large baking dish, combine the black pepper, salt, garlic, cumin, oregano, and lime juice. Pork (or lamb) tenderloin should be added to the baking dish with the lime juice and spice mixture, stirring to coat the meat. Refrigerate the baking dish covered. The pork (or lamb) should be marinated for at least 30 minutes, but ideally up to 2 hours.

Remove the pork (or lamb) from the baking dish and discard the marinade after marinating it. Grill the pork (or lamb) until a meat thermometer placed into the thickest part of the tenderloin reads 160 degrees, about 25 to 30 minutes (you may want to spray the rack with cooking spray to keep it from sticking)

Set aside for five minutes before slicing 1/4-inch thick. Garnish with green onions and cilantro, if desired.

Winter Squash Stuffed and Baked

Depending on the size of the squash and if it is served as a main dish or a side dish, this recipe will provide 6-8 serves.

Ingredients:

Squash, around a medium size (pumpkin or Hubbard work best, but any winter squash that you happen to have on hand will work fine for this recipe)

2 cups of brown rice that has been cooked (about 1 cup uncooked)

1 12 cups cranberries that are dried

1 cup of chicken or vegetable broth

1 cup chopped pecans

2 tablespoons of chopped fresh sage

Thime is 1 teaspoon per serving.

2 tablespoons of extra virgin olive oil

Ground flax seed, 2 tbsp (use flax seed meal or grind your own flax seeds) The salt content is 2 teaspoons.

Preparation:

As a first step, turn on your oven to 400 degrees Fahrenheit. Remove the seeds by cutting off the top of the winter squash (such as a pumpkin or Hubbard squash). In a large dish, combine the rest of the ingredients and then fill the winter squash. Replace the squash's top and brush it with a little olive oil before serving. Bake the squash for an hour or until it is tender enough to be pierced easily with a knife on a cookie sheet or baking dish.

After removing the squash from the oven, let it to cool for a few minutes before slicing and serving.

CPSIA information can be obtained
at www.ICGtesting.com
Printed in the USA
BVHW031212290722
643331BV00013B/306